CONTENTS

FATAL SILENCE?

Freedom of Expression and the Right to Health in Burma

ARTICLE 19
July 1996

ACKNOWLEDGEMENTS

This report was written by Martin Smith, a journalist and specialist writer on Burma and South East Asia.

ARTICLE 19 gratefully acknowledges the support of the Open Society Institute for this publication.

ARTICLE 19 would also like to acknowledge the considerable information, advice and constructive criticism supplied by very many different individuals and organisations working in the health and humanitarian fields on Burma. Such information was willingly supplied in the hope that it would increase both domestic and international understanding of the serious health problems in Burma. Under current political conditions, however, many aid workers have asked not to be identified.

© ARTICLE 19
ISBN 1 870798 13 9

"The enjoyment of the highest attainable standard of health is one of the fundamental rights of every human being without distinction of race, religion, political belief, economic or social conditions."

World Health Organization Constitution (Preamble)

ABBREVIATIONS

ABSDF	All Burma Students Democratic Front
AIDS	acquired immune deficiency syndrome
ASEAN	Association of South East Asian Nations
BADP	Border Areas Development Programme
BBC	British Broadcasting Corporation/Burmese Border Consortium
BPI	Burma Pharmaceutical Industry
BSPP	Burma Socialist Programme Party
CIA	Central Intelligence Agency
DKBO	Democratic Karen Buddhist Organization
HIV	human immunodeficiency virus
ICCPR	International Covenant on Civil and Political Rights
ICRC	International Committee of the Red Cross
IDU	intravenous drug user
ILO	International Labour Organization
IMR	infant mortality rate
KIO	Kachin Independence Organization
KNU	Karen National Union
KNPP	Karenni National Progressive Party
MMA	Myanmar Medical Association
MMCWA	Myanmar Maternal and Child Welfare Association
MNRC	Mon National Relief Committee
MP	Member of Parliament
MRC	Myanmar Red Cross
MSF	Médecins Sans Frontières
MTA	Mong Tai Army
NGO	non-governmental organization
NLD	National League for Democracy
SLORC	State Law and Order Restoration Council
STD	sexually-transmitted disease
UDHR	Universal Declaration of Human Rights
UN	United Nations
UNDP	United Nations Development Programme
UNDCP	United Nations International Drug Control Programme
UNHCR	United Nations High Commissioner for Refugees
UNICEF	United Nations Children's Fund
UNPFA	United Nations Population Fund
US	United States of America
USAID	United States Agency for International Development
USDA	Union Solidarity and Development Association
UWSP	United Wa State Party
WHO	World Health Organization

Chapter 1

OVERVIEW

Censorship has long concealed a multitude of grave issues in Burma (Myanmar[1]). After decades of governmental secrecy and isolation, Burma was dramatically thrust into world headlines during the short-lived democracy uprising in the summer of 1988. But, while international concern and pressure has since continued to mount over the country's long-standing political crisis, the health and humanitarian consequences of over 40 years of political malaise and ethnic conflict have largely been neglected. Indeed, in many parts of the country, they remain totally unaddressed.

There are many elements involved in addressing the health crisis which now besets Burma's peoples. A fundamental aspect, in ARTICLE 19's view, is for the rights to freedom of expression and information, together with the right to democratic participation, to be ensured. In a context of censorship and secrecy, individuals cannot make informed decisions on important matters affecting their health. Without freedom of academic research and the ability to disseminate research findings, there can be no informed public debate. Denial of research and information also makes effective health planning and provision less likely at the national level. Without local participation, founded on freedom of expression and access to information, the health needs of many sections of society are likely to remain unaddressed. Likewise, secrecy and censorship have a negative impact on the work of international humanitarian agencies.

Although not comparable to the crises in Rwanda or Somalia, modern-day Burma has one of the poorest health records and lowest standards of living in the developing world. At independence in 1948, the country was regarded as one of the most fertile and potentially prosperous lands in Asia. By the time of the democracy uprising in 1988, however, Burma had become one of the world's ten poorest nations. With an average per capita income of just US$ 250 per annum, today Burma is categorized by the United Nations (UN) as a Least Developed Country (LDC).

Fatal Silence?

Health statistics can be notoriously unreliable in Burma and, by selective quoting, very different pictures of the national health situation can be painted. With so little data available, health problems can be overestimated as well as underestimated. But among a plethora of urgent health issues, the following stand out as the legacies of decades of social and political neglect:

—   Burma currently has one of the highest rates of infant and
     maternal mortality in Asia;
—   only one third of the country has access to clean water or proper
     sanitation;
—   nearly half of all children of primary school age are
     malnourished;
—   with only one doctor for every 12,500 people, the national
     system of health care does not extend to even half the country;
—   health education is woefully inadequate, and only 25 per cent of
     all children complete the five basic years of primary school;
—   Burma is the world's largest producer of illicit opium and heroin,
     which has a grave health impact in both Burma and the
     international community at large;
—   HIV/AIDS is increasing at an alarming rate, with estimates of
     HIV-carriers increasing from near zero to 500,000 over the past
     six years;
—   Burma has generated over one million refugees or internally-
     displaced people as a result of civil war;
—   Burma has over one million inhabitants who have been
     compulsorily resettled by the government, whose health and
     living conditions are also often poor;
—   finally, it is treatable or preventable illnesses or conditions linked
     to poor socio-economic status, such as intestinal infestations,
     pneumonia, tuberculosis, malnutrition, malaria and
     complications arising from illicit abortions, which continue to
     be the main causes of unnecessary death and ill-suffering in the
     country.

Not surprisingly, in view of the scale of these problems, virtually all international agencies attempting to establish operations inside Burma since 1988 have chosen health and education programmes as their first point of entry. For far too long, Burma's health and humanitarian crises have been allowed to continue, virtually unacknowledged and unreported, under a stifling blanket of governmental censorship and inaction. Indeed, so alarmed were they by the results of new field-surveys that, in 1992, officials of the United Nations Children's Fund (UNICEF) considered calling for an urgent campaign of international humanitarian relief to alleviate what they described as "Myanmar's Silent Emergency":

> For a long time the state of Myanmar's children was perhaps one of the country's best kept secrets. Decades of self-imposed isolation, fabricated statistics and the absence of social research and journalistic inquiry had created a false image of social developments... . In fact, neither the outside world nor even the authorities inside Myanmar have an accurate or complete appreciation of the very serious conditions in the social sectors.[2]

While there can be little argument over humanitarian need, many medical practitioners in Burma nevertheless remain cautious about allowing the issue of health to be used as another battleground by different actors and institutions during the present political impasse. Under the military State Law and Order Restoration Council (SLORC), which assumed power in 1988, Burma has entered its third critical period of political and economic transition since independence in 1948. But, although the first international non-governmental organizations (NGOs) have been allowed to return under the SLORC's "open-door" economic policy[3], internal political repression has continued at a high level. In particular, the SLORC has never accepted the result of the 1990 general election, in which the National League for Democracy (NLD) won a landslide victory. Over the past eight years, thousands of democracy supporters and NLD activists, including the party's leader Daw Aung San Suu Kyi, have been detained without trial or sentenced to prison terms for peaceful opposition to the SLORC.[4]

In such a polarized atmosphere, the universal importance of human rights — including the right to health — frequently becomes lost amidst arguments over political or security priorities. Opposition groups, especially, have expressed grave doubts over the effectiveness and equity of new health programmes introduced by the SLORC. Without the rights and institutions inherent in a democratic society, they argue, any health impact will be necessarily limited and only related to projects that the military government approves. Moreover, such health projects will not address the many human rights violations, such as forced labour, forced relocations or summary arrests and imprisonment, which themselves have an extremely detrimental impact on the health of individuals. According to Dr Thaung Htun, health spokesperson for the National Coalition Government Union of Burma, which consists of eleven exiled MPs who won seats in the 1990 election:

> The humanitarian crisis in Burma today is a direct outcome of 33 years of military misrule. How can any humanitarian problems be tackled without first addressing the root problems which are political?[5]

By contrast, many other doctors and community leaders hope that health and development programmes will help create the social and political bonds necessary for rebuilding their long-divided societies after so many years of suffering and conflict. This view is most prevalent in ethnic minority regions of the country where cease-fires have recently been achieved by the SLORC with over a dozen armed ethnic opposition groups. According to this argument, the spirit of peace and social regeneration in the war zones will eventually break the political deadlock in Rangoon. "As long as there is peace, we believe the political discussions can continue," stated Major-General Zau Mai, chairman of the Kachin Independence Organization (KIO), which signed a cease-fire agreement with the SLORC in 1994.[6]

Despite such conciliatory words, however, the tasks of social and political reconstruction now facing Burma are enormous. At a time of widespread poverty and economic uncertainty for the majority of Burma's peoples, the entire health system is in a state of crisis, reflecting the many years of governmental inaction and political stagnation. Corruption and inefficiency are rife; censorship is pervasive; draconian political restrictions are enforced on all medical practitioners; health information is scarce and often inaccurate; and large areas of the country remain inaccessible to independent health workers and journalists. Indeed, while the first international NGOs and aid agencies were still tentatively returning to Burma, in June 1995 the International Committee of the Red Cross (ICRC) decided to pull out of Burma altogether in protest at continuing restrictions over monitoring the health of prisoners and the lack of governmental co-operation with its humanitarian work (see Chapter 6.3).

This report, therefore, highlights crucial issues of health and human rights in a society under censorship, at a time of historic transition. Since few studies have ever been published on the national health system in Burma, the first part examines the underlying issues of health and human rights against the backdrop of the country's long-running political malaise. The second part then looks at three specific areas of concern: humanitarian emergency, AIDS and narcotics, and women's health. Each topic raises fundamental issues over the rights of all people to freedom of expression, and to freedom of research and information.

In ARTICLE 19's view, these most fundamental of human rights are absolutely central to the provision and enjoyment of essential health care — which is itself a universal human right — in any country in the world.

NOTES

[1] Burma was renamed "Myanmar" by the State Law and Order Restoration Council (SLORC) government in 1989 as part of a governmental policy to change or re-transliterate many place names and titles. However, although recognized at the United Nations, the new term "Myanmar" is still rejected by most democratic and ethnic opposition parties.

[2] UNICEF, *Possibilities for a United Nations Peace and Development Initiative for Myanmar* (Draft for Consultation, 16 March 1992), 1. The UNICEF plan was abandoned after this document was leaked.

[3] During 1995, at least 15 NGOs had programmes or representatives in the country, most of which had entered Burma since 1994. Not all had Memoranda of Understanding and some later left or were rejected by the SLORC, but among NGOs reportedly represented in the country during the year were: Action Internationale Contre la Faim, Adventist Development and Relief Agency, Association Francois-Xavier Bagnoud, Australian Red Cross, Bridge

Asia Japan, Care International, Groupe de Recherche et d'Echanges Technologiques, International Committee of the Red Cross, International Federation of Eye Banks, International Federation of the Red Cross and Red Crescent Societies, Leprosy Mission International, Médecins du Monde, Médecins Sans Frontières (France and Netherlands), Population Services International, Sasakawa Foundation, Save the Children (UK), World Concern and World Vision International.

[4] The political events since 1988 have been examined more fully in ARTICLE 19, *State of Fear: Censorship in Burma* (London: 1991); ARTICLE 19, *Paradise Lost? The Suppression of Environmental Rights and Freedom of Expression in Burma* (London:1994); and ARTICLE 19, *Censorship Prevails: Political Deadlock and Economic Transition in Burma* (London: 1995).

[5] Interview, 23 May 1995.

[6] Interview, 7 April 1994.

Chapter 2

HEALTH RIGHTS AND HUMAN RIGHTS
The Experience of Burma

Burma today presents an acute example of the vital link between the realization of the right to health, freedom of expression and the protection of other human rights. Among international development organizations, research and analysis into this fundamental interdependence are still evolving: many of the ethical issues raised by modern science or public health law and practice are extremely complex. Nevertheless, although not always explicitly stated, the basic "right to health" has long been enshrined in a number of international human rights declarations and treaties. Pre-eminent among these is Article 25 of the Universal Declaration of Human Rights (UDHR), which states:

> Everyone has the right to a standard of living adequate for the health and well-being of himself and his family, including food, clothing, housing and medical care and the right to security in the event of unemployment, sickness, disability, widowhood, old age or other lack of livelihood in circumstances beyond his control.

In addition, other provisions of the UDHR have a bearing on health. Article 3 guarantees "the right to life, liberty and security of person", while Article 5 provides that "no one shall be subjected to torture, or to cruel, inhuman or degrading treatment or punishment".[1]

Based upon such fundamental tenets of human rights, over the years a number of other human rights instruments have been adopted by governments which explicitly recognize a universal right to health. Some agreements relate to specific human rights violations, such as the 1987 Convention Against Torture and Other Cruel, Inhuman or Degrading Treatment or Punishment. Other health guarantees are contained in treaties that are intended to protect disadvantaged or particular social groups. For example, the right to

7

health is invoked in Article 5 of the 1969 Convention on the Elimination of All Forms of Racial Discrimination, Articles 11 and 12 of the 1981 Convention on the Elimination of All Forms of Discrimination Against Women, and Article 24 of the 1989 Convention on the Rights of the Child.

In practice, however, for doctors and other health practitioners working in the field, recent research has suggested that medical and ethical concerns over health and human rights violations generally fall into two main categories.[2] The first is the grievous impact that many human rights violations have on health, including such gross violations as torture, extrajudicial execution, rape, forcible resettlement or forced labour.[3] Whether administering to victims or addressing the humanitarian impact of war, health practitioners are frequently principal witnesses to the suffering and are thrust into the front line of care.

The second key area of concern is equally critical: the impact that government policies and public health programmes or practices themselves have on health and other human rights. In this approach, it is recognized that the fundamental issue of health care cannot be isolated from human rights more generally or from overall social conditions. The broad social basis of the right to health was most clearly stated in the historic Alma-Ata Declaration of the World Health Organization (WHO) and UNICEF, which was adopted at the International Conference on Primary Health Care in 1978:

> The Conference strongly reaffirms that health, which is a state of complete physical, mental and social well-being, and not merely the absence of disease or infirmity, is a fundamental human right and that the attainment of the highest possible level of health is a most important world-wide social goal whose realisation requires the action of many other social and economic sectors in addition to the health sector.

In recent years, the World Bank, too, has emphasized the detrimental impact of poverty on the health of people in developing countries and required governments to "pursue sound macroeconomic policies that emphasize reduction of poverty" as a "central" means of achieving "good health".[4]

In line with such arguments, it is today taken as axiomatic by a growing number of international development agencies and governments that the proper assessment, development and implementation of equitable health programmes in response to the humanitarian and social needs of the community is a central responsibility of any government. By contrast, failure to provide accessible health care, discrimination against women or minority ethnic or religious groups in the provision of health care, ill-treatment of prison inmates, or failure to provide adequate programmes in vital health areas, such as maternal welfare or HIV/AIDS, can all constitute the most fundamental violations of human rights.

A crucial aspect of this broad approach to the right to health is the increased emphasis placed on preventive aspects of health care rather than on medical treatment itself, a trend also advocated by the World Bank.[5] According to WHO estimates, for example, half a million women die around the world every year from avoidable pregnancy-related causes, of whom 90 per cent live in developing countries.[6] Similarly, as Médecins Sans Frontières (MSF), a leading NGO in the health field, has pointed out, the great majority of deaths occurring in children under five each year are "avoidable mortality": that is, deaths from preventable or treatable illnesses, such as malaria, diarrhoea, measles, malnutrition or respiratory infections.[7]

For this reason, the Plan of Action adopted by the 1990 UN World Summit for Children targeted the "health, nutrition and education of women" as the key to reducing the shockingly high rates of both maternal and infant mortality in many parts of the developing world. Indeed, access to information and the right to know, which are guaranteed in Article 19 of the Universal Declaration of Human Rights, constitute a vital basis of preventive health care.[8] Communities and citizens need basic information to make informed choices over everyday health issues such as birth spacing, for example, as well as to understand how they can avoid the risks of illnesses such as HIV/AIDS or cholera.

At the same time, for the supply of such information to be truly effective, providing public access to health care is not enough. The right of public participation, which is also stated in the UN

Declaration on the Right to Development[9], must be guaranteed in an accountable system of health management, where independent data collection and efficient monitoring of health programmes and practices are permitted as democratic rights. As with many other health failings in the country, the denial of such a system is a problem not only confined to Burma. Over the years, as a recent investigation by ARTICLE 19 into reproductive health pointed out, many governments around the world have been able to "manipulate, suppress or fail to provide information", which has contributed to the ill-health or deaths of millions of people.[10]

Starvation, disease, poverty, injury, genocide and other gross human rights violations arising out of armed conflict are perhaps the most extreme health emergencies that, all too frequently, have been concealed by censorship. But a host of other grave health issues also threaten the state of global health and continue to be under-documented and under-reported, from the pandemic spread of HIV/AIDS and the resurgence of tuberculosis in the past 15 years to reproductive health issues and other such perennial problems as drug abuse, cholera and malaria. Yet, despite this bleak picture, many physicians are confident that a growing number of health problems — including virtually all infectious or parasitic diseases — are either controllable or can be prevented altogether by a combination of education, access to information, diagnostic capacity, the availability of modern medicines and treatment, and the financing of relevant health programmes.[11]

Tragically, although Burma represents an outstanding example of the need to respect a broad range of human rights in order to protect health rights, substantive debate on these issues has scarcely begun. Burma today is suffering the consequences of five decades of political confrontation and over 30 years of military rule.

Many of the gravest issues affecting the health of Burma's peoples result from armed conflict. Since 1988, such inhumane practices as torture, extrajudicial executions and "scorched earth" tactics by the government have been documented by international human rights organizations and given considerable publicity abroad (see Chapter 6.1). In this context, it should be noted that armed opposition groups have also, over the years, been responsible for many gross abuses that have had a negative impact on health and inhibited the development of more equitable systems of public health care.

In recent years, however, the sufferings of the Burmese peoples have undoubtedly been compounded by the government's social and economic reforms. For while the SLORC's "market-oriented", "open-door" economic policies have clearly brought new prosperity to certain sectors of the community (especially traders and families of the ruling elite), a growing number of health problems have been observed by medical practitioners in different regions of the country. Opposition groups argue that the SLORC's economic and development reforms have been ill-planned, discriminatory and often simply exploitative, causing many families to lose their traditional livelihoods or lands.[12] For example, many doctors believe that, in several parts of Burma, the continuing high incidence of such serious health problems as malnutrition, malaria, diarrhoea and various water-borne diseases can be directly attributed to governmental policies of civilian resettlement or "forced relocations" under various development or counter-insurgency programmes. Indeed, since the SLORC assumed power in 1988, over one million people are estimated to have been forcibly relocated in the countryside or moved from downtown urban areas to new satellite towns around Rangoon and other main conurbations (see Chapter 6.2). In some rural relocation sites, health workers have found over 50 per cent of children under five to be suffering from malnutrition. Along with poor sanitation and inadequate health infrastructures, malnutrition is a major, though largely unreported, factor behind the high rates of infant mortality in many communities.

On the national scale, UNICEF has also recorded a recent rise in malnutrition among children under three from 32.4 per cent in 1990 to 36.66 per cent in 1991 (including a rise from 9.2 to 11.19 per cent severely malnourished), and in 1991 raised the estimated prevalency rate of stunting among school beginners (which is indicative of past or chronic malnutrition) from 29.1 to 40.5 per cent.[13] The consequences of such nutritional neglect can also be detected in the nationally high rates of Vitamin A and iodine deficiency, which lead to poor physical and cognitive development. For example, UNICEF considers a goitre prevalency rate (caused by lack of iodine) of more than five per cent a "public health threat", but among schoolchildren in the Chin State a rate as high as 65 per cent has been recorded.[14]

Some of the most extreme examples of new health problems in Burma today can be seen in the boom town mining communities of the

Kachin and Shan States, where hundreds of thousands of people from all over the country have rushed in the past few years in the hope of striking it rich. In the malaria-infested jade-mining region at Hpakhan or the ruby mines at Mongshu, some doctors have made private fortunes providing personal health care for those who can pay, but for most local inhabitants there is little health provision at all. For many years, foreign journalists and international health organizations have been barred from all such sensitive regions of the country. But recent travellers report that intravenous drug use, prostitution and the closely-attendant spread of HIV/AIDS are all flourishing against a deadly backdrop of ignorance and social crisis that desperately reflects the changing pressures and patterns in modern life.

In contrast to this evidence of neglect, since assuming power in 1988 the SLORC has belatedly shown some awareness of the responsibilities of government for the protection of health rights in Burma. Prior to 1988, under General Ne Win's isolationist "Burmese Way to Socialism", Burma was one of the world's most reticent signatories to international agreements and conventions. However, in one of many ambivalent steps taken by the ruling generals, from 1989 the SLORC government began to sign or acknowledge a broad array of international conventions. Prominent among these are the 1949 Geneva Conventions, the UN Convention on the Rights of the Child, the World Declaration for Nutrition, the Vienna Convention for the Protection of the Ozone Layer, and the UN Convention Against Illicit Traffic in Narcotic Drugs and Psychotropic Substances, all of which contain important provisions relating to health and humanitarian issues.[15] In addition, the SLORC has for the first time entered Burma into a number of agreements that include other important health provisions with different international agencies or countries, including the UN International Drug Control Programme (UNDCP), the UN High Commissioner for Refugees (UNHCR), China, Thailand and Bangladesh.

Domestically, too, the SLORC has appeared to show greater interest in addressing certain health issues than did its predecessor, the Burma Socialist Programme Party (BSPP) government of General Ne Win (1962-1988). A number of basic health rights had been officially recognized under the BSPP's 1974 Constitution, including the "right to medical treatment" (Article 149), the "right to rest and recreation" (Article 150), the right to "enjoy benefits for injury due to occupational accidents or when disabled or sick or old" (Article 151), and "equal rights for women" (Article 154). The 1974 Constitution has been suspended since 1988. However, both the duties of government and the rights of the people to information and participation appear to have been further recognized at the National Convention in Rangoon, which the SLORC convened in 1993 to draft a new constitution. This would appear evident from the 104 basic principles that have been drafted to date — for example, Principle 18 (a) and (b) declares: "The State shall earnestly strive to improve the education and health of the people; the State shall enact necessary law to enable the national people to participate in matters of education and health of the people."[16]

The actual timetable for introducing Burma's new constitution is contentious and uncertain. In November 1995, the NLD officially withdrew from the Convention in public protest at the many political restrictions and the lack of "freedom of discussion"; the Convention, Aung San Suu Kyi said, did not represent "the will of the people".[17] The SLORC, nevertheless, has continued to convene sessions of the Convention without the participation of the NLD, which has also been barred by the SLORC from further attendance.

Although the political process remains deadlocked, the SLORC has, over the past few years, taken some steps to introduce social and economic reforms. In the health field, a National Health Committee has been set up under the SLORC Secretary-One, Lieutenant-General Khin Nyunt, to co-ordinate activities between the different government ministries and health departments. In the language of their deliberations, the influence of different UN agencies is often clear. The cornerstone of current health policy is Burma's National Health Plan 1993-96, which is based upon the goals of the WHO's "Health For All by the year 2,000". To support these objectives, a number of specialist programmes have also been set up, including the National Drug Policy (1991), National Population Policy (1992), National Health Policy (1993), National Programme of Action for the Survival, Protection and Development of Myanmar's Children in the 1990s (1993), and the National Plan of Action for Food and Nutrition (1994). Important targets in the National Programme of Action for Children, for example, are the halving of the rates of both infant and maternal mortality, immunization of 90 per cent of all infants, and provision of "access to information about and preventive measures against HIV/ AIDS to all at-risk groups".[18] In another significant development, NGO and community-based approaches to health have also been proposed (see Chapter 3).

And yet, despite the declaration of such important goals, many medical practitioners and international aid agencies contend that the overall health and humanitarian situation in Burma has either not improved or has actually gone from bad to worse over the past decade. The ICRC's withdrawal from Burma in June 1995 was perhaps the sharpest indication of international concern over the government's approach to health and humanitarian issues in practice (see Chapter 6.3). All Western bilateral aid to Burma was also cut off in 1988 in protest at the violent manner of the SLORC's assumption of power. Then, in May 1992, in response to human rights concerns that aid was not reaching the people, the Governing Council of the UN Development Programme (UNDP) took the extraordinary decision to halt new funding for its Burma Country Programme for one year until a complete review had been undertaken to ensure that future projects would reach the "grass-roots level" in a "sustainable manner".[19] The result of these deliberations was the formulation of the UNDP's "Human Development Initiative" for Burma, which aims to improve the " people's welfare through participatory development involving communities and grass-roots initiatives".[20]

But, undoubtedly the most serious humanitarian questions have been raised by the continuing work of the UN Commission on Human Rights and its Special Rapporteur to Myanmar. In a series of reports published since 1992, the Special Rapporteur has documented a disturbing background of gross human rights violations, all of which would have contributed to the poor health environment in the country, despite the recent spread of cease-fires between the SLORC and armed ethnic opposition groups. For example, while welcoming the release of Aung San Suu Kyi in July 1995, the Special Rapporteur's most recent statement to the UN General Assembly cited continuing evidence of summary executions, arbitrary detentions, torture, rape, forced relocations, forced labour for government development projects and forced porterage, in which conscripted citizens are compelled to work in "appalling living conditions".[21] The SLORC's formal health policies absolutely fail to address the impact of human rights violations of this kind on the population's health.

On 5 December 1995 the UN General Assembly also demonstrated its continuing concern about a wide range of human rights and humanitarian issues when it urged the SLORC, by consensus resolution, to "ensure full respect for human rights and fundamental freedoms, including freedom of expression and assembly", as well as to "put an end to violations of the right to life and integrity of the human being" (Clause 11). In January 1996, too, the European Commission declared it had received sufficient allegations of human rights violations that are contrary to International Labour Organization (ILO) Conventions and "International Humanitarian Law" to begin a formal investigation into forced labour in Burma, with a view to suspending economic tariff privileges under the European Union's Generalized Scheme of Preferences.[22]

However, despite this growing body of international evidence and condemnation, the SLORC has continued to reject all criticism and deny any wrongdoing. Like certain other Asian governments facing international criticism over their violations of civil and political rights, the SLORC chooses to invoke a different definition of human rights, a definition that gives far greater priority to the collective economic and social well-being of the population in general rather than respect for the basic human rights of individuals. Speaking at the University for Development of National Races in February 1995, Senior General Than Shwe, the SLORC Chairman, described the relationship between different human rights in the following terms:

> It is regarded that food, clothing and shelter needs
> are the most basic human rights for mankind to
> survive. It can be said that once the basic human
> rights of the people are met, there is no difficulty
> to fulfil other human rights.[23]

Such arguments have also been advanced by SLORC officials in the international community. According to U Aung Aye, who led the Myanmar delegation at the 51st session of the UN Commission on Human Rights in March 1994:

> Human rights cannot be enjoyed in a vacuum....
> Our concept of justice is not only justice in its le-
> gal sense but also social, economic and political
> justice.

Few observers would disagree that there is a close interdependence between social and economic rights and civil and political rights. Indeed, one argument made in this report is that violations of a wide range of human rights — including freedom of expression and information, torture, extrajudicial execution and forced labour — have an important bearing on the health of the population. Yet, to date, the SLORC has steadfastly refused to investigate any specific reports of human rights violations, despite the repeated criticisms of the UN General Assembly. In its most recent reply to the UN Special Rapporteur to Myanmar, the SLORC simply dismissed all his allegations as "unfounded, emanating from anti-government sources and terrorist groups, with the aim of discrediting the Government as well as the Armed Forces of Myanmar".[24]

It would thus appear that, although all sides in Burma publicly say they recognize the need for social and political reform, for the moment freedom of expression and the important linkage between health rights and other human rights are not even on the national agenda.

NOTES

[1] These universal rights to life or health are further guaranteed in both the International Covenant on Civil and Political Rights (ICCPR) (e.g., Art. 6.1) and the International Covenant on Economic, Social and Cultural Rights (Art. 12.1).

[2] See, J M Mann et al., "Health and Human Rights", in *1 (1) Health and Human Rights* (Fall 1994), 6-23; and V A Leary, "The Right to Health in International Human Rights Law", ibid., at 24-56. Many doctors and aid specialists would also make a further distinction between "health" and "medicine", the latter being only one factor in the former. For example, although political will is clearly needed to improve any system of national health care, doctors can often alleviate individual suffering or illness by providing immediate medical treatment, regardless of the wider political or health contexts, as long as access is allowed.

16

[3] Mann et al., note 2 above, at 17.

[4] The World Bank, *World Development Report 1993* (Oxford University Press: 1993), 6.

[5] Ibid., at 6-7.

[6] ARTICLE 19, *The Right to Know: Human Rights and Access to Reproductive Health Information* (London and Philadelphia: ARTICLE 19 and University of Pennsylvania Press, 1995), 88.

[7] Médecins Sans Frontières, *Populations in Danger 1995* (London: MSF, 1995), 118. Many doctors would question whether malaria, which shows considerable drug resistance, is truly preventable or treatable. Virulent strains of falciparum malaria, in particular, are endemic in Burma's borderland areas. Nevertheless, in contrast to most of its neighbours, negligible progress has been made in combating this often fatal sickness which modern treatments can greatly alleviate.

[8] Article 19: "Everyone has the right to freedom of opinion and expression; this right includes freedom to hold opinions without interference and to seek, receive and impart information and ideas through any media and regardless of frontiers."

[9] UN Declaration on the Right to Development (1986), Art. 2.3: "States have the right and the duty to formulate appropriate national development policies that aim at the constant improvement of the well-being of the entire population and of all individuals, on the basis of their active, free and meaningful participation in development and in the fair distribution of the benefits resulting therefrom."

[10] ARTICLE 19, note 6 above, at 72.

[11] MSF, note 7 above, at 121.

[12] Since shortly after the 1990 election, the NLD has been forbidden from bringing out any new publications. For the NLD's economic manifesto and an interview on the subject with Aung San Suu Kyi, see, *Sunday Morning Post* (Hong Kong), 14 April 1996.

[13] UNICEF, *Children and Women in Myanmar: A Situation Analysis 1995* (Rangoon: 1995), 27 and 31.

[14] Ibid.

[15] The SLORC, however, has not ratified either the ICCPR or the International Covenant on Economic, Social and Cultural Rights which, together with the UDHR, comprise the International Bill of Human Rights.

[16] Further principles in the proposed constitution concern the provision of health care by the state for mothers, children, orphans, the families of fallen army servicemen, and the aged or disabled, as well as the expansion of both the private and public medical sectors.

[17] Reuters, 29 Nov. 1995; see also, ARTICLE 19, *Censorship Prevails* (see Chapter 1, note 4), 25-29.

[18] *National Programme of Action for the Survival, Protection and Development of Myanmar's Children in the 1990s* (Rangoon: 1993), 6.

[19] See UNDP, *Summary Report: UNDP Assistance to Myanmar (as per GC decision 93/21)* (Rangoon: May 1995).

[20] C A Serrato, *Targeting Development Assistance to the Lowest-Income Populations of Myanmar: A Report to the United Nations Development Programme* (UNDP, Rangoon: 1995), 2. See also, Chapter 9.

[21] UN General Assembly, *Situation of Human Rights in Myanmar: Note by the Secretary-General* (New York, A/50/568, 16 Oct. 1995), 17.

[22] European Commission, *Initiation of an Investigation of Forced Labour Practices in Myanmar* (Brussels, IP/96/44,16 Jan. 1996).

[23] *New Light of Myanmar,* 11 Feb. 1995.

[24] UN General Assembly, note 21 above, at 31.

Chapter 3

THE HEALTH SYSTEM IN BURMA

As in other state sectors, there has long been a yawning gap between the reality and rhetoric concerning the provision of health care nationally in Burma. Few independent studies have ever been permitted and, until the recent cease-fires between the government and armed ethnic opposition groups, many regions of the country had remained strictly off-limits to international observers for decades. Even today, vast areas remain either officially forbidden or are inaccessible to outside agencies, especially in the ethnic minority states.

In the absence of other sources of information, health analysts have been largely dependent on official government reports and statistics which, ever since General Ne Win seized power in 1962, have consistently depicted an expanding and progressive medical system. On paper at least, a comprehensive health system was built up during the BSPP era with large hospitals, dispensaries and a variety of specialist health centres in the main towns of all of Burma's 14 states and divisions, as well as a system of local co-operatives.[1] Smaller hospitals and facilities were also developed, including maternal and child health centres, under the supervision of a qualified Medical Officer in each of the country's 319 local townships. Privately, however, government doctors admit that effective health provision never extended to much more than a third of the country. In part, this was due to governmental neglect and lack of resources. But it was also due, in large part, to the insurgencies. Even today it is still possible to find nurses and other health workers drawing government salaries in military garrison towns, who have never travelled into the countryside to take up their positions.[2]

Since 1988, in response to the SLORC's moves towards a "market-oriented" economy, a number of new initiatives have been mooted by government servants in the Ministry of Health. Many of these would appear to mark a distinct break with the past. Emphasis, for example, is now officially given to the role of "community organizations", the return of foreign NGOs to Burma, and increased co-operation with different UN agencies.[3]

However, as opposition groups point out, many of the structural mechanisms and working practices from the BSPP era have been maintained. The BSPP's third "People's Health Plan" of 1986-1990, for example, continued uninterrupted by the momentous events of Burma's "democracy summer" in 1988, and in 1991 was replaced by a series of new "National Health Plans", which followed virtually the same goals. An updated and more relevant National Health Policy was promulgated in 1993 (see Chapter 2), but — as in other walks of national life — doctors complain that military control over the top echelons of decision-making remains absolute. In consequence, the Health Ministry, which is headed by Vice-Admiral Than Nyunt, remains highly bureaucratic and slow to respond to the needs of the people. Indeed, much of the energy and influence behind recent changes comes not from the Ministry but from the National Health Committee, a powerful inter-ministerial grouping which is chaired by Lieutenant-General Khin Nyunt, the SLORC Secretary-One and head of the Military Intelligence Service. As an indication of the concentration of power in a few individuals in Burma, Khin Nyunt, who is regarded in ruling circles as a progressive within the SLORC on development issues, also chairs the government's Education, Foreign Affairs, Tourism and Border Areas Development Committees. Like Vice-Admiral Than Nyunt, however, Khin Nyunt is believed to have no formal medical experience or training.

Despite a legacy of such inertia and military control, there can be little doubt that the growing involvement of foreign aid workers in Burma since 1988 has given a long overdue boost to the domestic and international recognition of serious health problems in the country. This has come about both by the continuing work of different UN agencies, which remained in Burma after the SLORC's assumption of power in 1988, as well as the arrival of the first international NGOs after 1991. In particular, following the SLORC's accession to the UN protocols on the Rights of the Child and the Geneva Conventions, the language appearing in official health reports has begun to fit more closely with international norms. However, it should be emphasized that the important ideals which are expressed in such reports come nowhere near describing the reality of human suffering or lack of adequate health or medical provision that exists in many parts of the country today.

Many of Burma's health problems are long-standing and can be dated back to previous governments. But medical workers in the field generally concur that, despite the publicity given to recent initiatives by UN agencies and foreign NGOs (especially relating to HIV/AIDS), for the majority of Burma's peoples both the health pressures and difficulties in finding access to adequate health treatment have increased since 1988 as the existing state system has begun to unravel.

In many respects, Burma today displays the classic characteristics of "strong societies" but a "weak state", where the authorities have been unable to achieve — or countenance — effective action across all social and ethnic sectors.[4] In government-controlled areas, there are, in fact, four different — although overlapping — systems of health provision: public, private, traditional (or indigenous) and military. But it is the public sector, upon which most urban inhabitants depend and which had, in theory, been freely available to all, that has come under the greatest pressures since 1988 and which is losing patients most rapidly to the other sectors.

The political pressures in the state sector are examined below (see Chapter 5), but health workers point to two major areas of failure which permeate every region of the country: chronic under-funding, and a neglect of health education and the preventive aspects of health care. Many of the most obvious failings can be seen in government hospitals. As one international health worker privately explained to ARTICLE 19: "Unless you have money, public hospitals are the next step to the grave."

Burma still has many committed doctors and nurses, and there are many everyday examples of philanthropy. Many honest and hard-working practitioners are also very sensitive to criticism about health issues in Burma over which they feel they have no control. Nevertheless, after years of under-funding and poor management, corruption has become endemic in the public health system, with patients often required to pay bribes or fees every step of the way — sometimes from the hospital gateman to even getting a bed. Essential medicines, too, are always in short supply, and for many years even those medicines which do arrive in the clinics and surgeries have been routinely, but illegally, sold off to black market or privately-run pharmacies that can be found in streets around many main hospitals. Although treatment is technically free, patients have been required to buy back from the pharmacies all medicines (and even cotton wool) that are needed for operations. In private, many hospital staff have freely acknowledged their involvement in such illegal sales; it is unpopular, for example, to be posted to work in hospital blood banks, since there is no access to medicines that can be sold. But in their defence, public health workers argue that their families simply cannot survive without raising extra sources of income. Doctors, for example, who are at the top of the public pay scale, have average salaries of just 1,500 kyats (US$ 15) per month.[5]

As a result, over the years there has been a constant exodus of qualified doctors from the public sector — either to go abroad or, more recently, into other occupations or into private medical practice in Burma. Throughout the country, despite a general expansion in primary health care over the past decade, there are huge gaps and constant interruptions in medical provision, making it difficult to sustain community health programmes. According to UNICEF, of Burma's 13,392 qualified doctors in 1993, only 4,998 were recorded in public service; the remaining 8,394 were working as general practitioners in the private (or co-operative[6]) sector; significantly, too, an estimated 80 per cent of government doctors also run private clinics, sometimes even during duty hours when they fail to turn up for their official work.[7] There is also serious under-staffing of other medical personnel, including midwives and nurses, and the former BSPP's Community Health Worker programme, which had given rudimentary training to over 30,000 volunteers, was recently discontinued.[8]

As Burma's 46 million population continues to grow rapidly, these changing working practices and health demands have led to a very disparate level in the quality of health provision around the country. In January 1995, in a rare admission of problems, health officials privately reported that 500 government health posts were vacant.[9] The situation is particularly acute in ethnic minority areas. During 1995, for example, a third of the 150 positions for doctors in the Rakhine State were reportedly unfilled. Although it is technically difficult to resign from such posts, in ethnic minority areas many physicians from other areas either do not turn up for work or simply apply for transfer on their day of arrival rather than remain in what are widely regarded as hardship postings with few career prospects. Indeed, so serious are current shortages of doctors that in January 1995 the SLORC introduced regulations by decree, compelling all medical graduates to work in the state system for a minimum of three years before requests to resign or travel abroad will be considered. This, however, has not stopped the exodus.

Against this background, the second health sector in Burma — the private sector — is booming and provides an increasingly broad range of health care. Because of the lack of resources in the public sector, many people automatically turn to the private sector first, where many doctors have established reputations or moonlight from their state jobs. Indeed, many government doctors simply refer patients to their private clinics if they want speedy treatment — and if they are able to pay. In Burma's convulsive economy, the charges can be astronomical: in the private sector a hysterectomy operation can cost 30,000 kyats, for example, which is twice the official annual wages of most state workers. Nonetheless, the new class of rising rich in Burma, especially traders or those with access to foreign exchange, are able to afford such prices, as is evident from the recent fashion in certain business circles for expensive "poly-clinics" with private rooms and air-conditioning. With Burma promoting 1996 as its "Year of the Tourist", private physicians have similarly begun to target the health concerns of foreigners, and in October 1995 the first 24-hour international clinic was opened in Rangoon by the Singapore-based AEA medical centre chain.

Concerns over the methods of private doctors are, in general, more to do with the equity and ethics of treatment than with its quality, which remains relatively high (see Chapter 4). This is also largely the case with the third main health sector in Burma, the traditional or indigenous, which also works in the private market. There has long been a consensus that traditional practices, including homeopathic and Chinese herbal medicine, have a worthy place in the overall scheme of treatments available in Burma. The Health Ministry, for example, has a Department of Traditional Medicine[10], and over the years UNICEF has run training programmes to try and equip traditional birth attendants (known as *lethe*) with additional skills and knowledge, especially about hygiene and nutrition.

However, over the past decade many doctors have become increasingly concerned over the numbers of untrained "quacks" operating on the fringes of modern medicine and the private market, who use the failures in the national health system to take advantage of the sick and needy. In Burma, virtually anyone can set up as a private or independent health practitioner. As a result, across the country there are thousands of self-appointed medics masquerading as private medical experts, who give injections and every kind of fake or inappropriate treatment. By some estimates, they number at least one to each of Burma's 60,000 villages. On some occasions, such practitioners are preferred by local custom, but more often than not their main selling point is their quick availability and deceptive self-promotion when compared to public or properly-qualified private doctors.

The tragedy, as many hospitals in Burma have witnessed, is that patients suffering from emergency conditions, such as snake-bites or cerebral malaria, are often only brought in after life-saving time has already been wasted on such imposters by impoverished families who, in addition, have wasted their money. Many such practitioners have picked up titbits of health terminology during military service or during training as community health volunteers, and they are thus able to persuade their victims. In vast rural areas of Burma, however, there is no system of health information or reporting which would allow such very basic issues to be addressed. Moreover, even where deaths have occurred through obvious maltreatment, many physicians complain that there is no compulsion or incentive within the existing public health system to investigate such blatant health rights abuses, even though relevant mechanisms reportedly exist.

By contrast, the final health sector in Burma, that of the Burmese Armed Forces or *Tatmadaw*, has remained largely impervious to the social upheavals of the past decade. Military hospitals are well-supplied with medicines and most have modern equipment. In addition to two large Defence Services hospitals in Rangoon, there are also military hospitals in Mandalay, Maymyo, Meiktila and other important regional towns, which in the last few years have been equipped with computerized blood-testing and other expensive machinery. For many years, an estimated 50 newly-graduated doctors have been conscripted annually for a three-year period of service with the *Tatmadaw*, often in dangerous front-line areas. However, some doctors do also volunteer for appointments to military hospitals, since not only are working conditions more favourable but there are also greater career possibilities for research and specialism. Brigadier Kyaw Win, for example, who was formally General Ne Win's personal physician, was widely regarded as one of Asia's top malariologists before his recent posting as Ambassador to Canada. In addition, the SLORC has established a Defence Services Medical College in Rangoon, where many sons and daughters of military officers have gained admission. As a result, doctors in the public health system privately say that, just as in the former BSPP era, senior military officers are becoming ever more institutionalized and far removed from the daily health sufferings of most ordinary people.

Nevertheless, despite better provisioning in the military health sector overall, many soldiers in the ranks privately complain that military health care is not evenly spread and does not always extend to their families. Malaria, for example, continues to inflict a steady casualty rate among young soldiers stationed in the war zones, with dozens of fatalities annually. Although soldiers are supposed to be supplied with prophylactic medicines, both health education and testing facilities in the field are often extremely poor.

In summary, then, all four sectors within the national health system face a host of critical problems during an era of social uncertainty and political transition, which many doctors and health workers are only too anxious to address. Many doctors, for example, believe that it is impossible to tackle properly such everyday health problems as malaria, AIDS or tuberculosis while so many different and unrelated medical practices or systems exist around the country. In addition to the problems of diagnosis and treatment, drug resistance and infection can very quickly spread.

Very belatedly, the need for new strategies and effective integration between the different sectors was apparently recognized by the Health Ministry in the 1993 National Health Policy. Although dismissed by opposition groups as government public relations, this pledged in Clause 5 to augment "the role of co-operative, joint ventures, private sectors and non-governmental organizations in delivery of health care in view of the changing economic system". In another overdue recognition of need, Clause 12 of the National Health Policy also promised to expand national health services for the first time to the border areas, following the cease-fires agreed between armed ethnic minority groups and the government (Chapter 6.1).

Then, in another policy shift in September 1994, the SLORC took the first steps towards abolishing the system of theoretically free health care that had existed in Burma under successive governments since independence. Recognizing the worsening resource constraints within the existing system, a new "cost-sharing system" was announced for the country's 717 state-run hospitals[11], 1,424 rural health centres, 306 dispensaries and 353 maternal and child health centres to enable the public sector to raise income locally and compete more effectively with the burgeoning private market. "The community financing or community cost-sharing is just a precursor of health insurance and social security schemes of the United States and European countries," one senior health official claimed.[12]

In essence, the new scheme consists of a list of 23 items and medicines that local health authorities can sell to raise revenue to subsidize other treatment and running costs. Typically, however, the new system has yet to be properly explained to health workers or reported in the state-controlled media to the general public. As a result, different prices and practices have been introduced in different hospitals in different parts of the country, causing many doctors to over-prescribe drugs which may be unsuitable but are plentiful (because they are on the list), while more apposite cures are unavailable. The concept of charges also appears to be becoming mandatory, with a Caesarean operation, for example, now costing 6,000-8,000 kyats in many hospitals after all the necessary medicines and materials have been purchased, leaving many poor families with the bleak choice between the possible death of a loved one or bankruptcy. Equally serious, this emphasis on revenue and costing within the health system continues to push doctors in the more lucrative direction of treatment and the curative aspects of medicine rather than education or preventive health care.

Access to medical treatment is, of course, essential, but many doctors and health workers maintain that education is the cheapest but most neglected health reform that is needed in Burma today. For such a reorientation to be effective, the peoples of Burma must themselves be mobilized to value the importance of health education after decades of governmental failings and neglect. However, whether such essential reforms can be initiated during the present state of political deadlock and crisis is very far from certain.

NOTES

[1] Organized under the Ministry of Co-operatives, local co-operative societies in the townships were initially used for the sale of rice, cooking oil, medicines and other rationed goods. After 1972, many were also encouraged to open clinics and employ doctors under a semi-subsidized, fee-paying system.

[2] This report does not specifically examine the provision of health care by armed opposition groups in the large areas of territory they control around Burma's borderlands. Many run their own health programmes but, in comparison to overall needs, such projects must be considered very small (see also, Chapter 6.2).

[3] Ministry of Health, *Union of Myanmar: National Health Plan (1993-1996)* (Rangoon: 1993), 2.

[4] See e.g., J Migdal, *Strong Societies and Weak States: State-Society Relations and State Capabilities in the Third World* (Princeton University Press, 1988).

[5] Providing accurate conversion rates is difficult in Burma. The official exchange rate of US$ 1 = 6 kyats is unrealistic and in no way compares with the market rate of US$ 1 = 100 kyats that is used in the streets; see, World Bank, *Myanmar: Policies for Sustaining Economic Reform* (New York: 16 Oct. 1995), 18-23, 27-32.

[6] Since 1988, the BSPP's co-operative health clinics have, in effect, moved into the private market but continue to be competitive by importing and diversifying their activities while still receiving subsidized medicines and goods.

[7] UNICEF, *Children and Women in Myanmar* (see Chapter 2, note 13), 50.

[8] In 1995 Burma had just 7,033 public nurses, 2,671 private nurses, 8,724 midwives, 1,682 Lady Health Visitors and 1,327 Health Assistants, most of whom were working at the community level; see, Union of Myanmar, *Review of the Financial, Economic and Social Conditions for 1994/95* (Rangoon: Ministry of National Planning and Economic Development, 1995), 196. Under another volunteer scheme begun in 1978, there were also an estimated 20,000 auxiliary midwives.

[9] *Bangkok Post*, 30 Jan. 1995.

[10] In addition to Traditional Medicine, there are four other main departments under the Ministry: Health, Medical Education, Medical Research and

Medical Statistics. Until the late 1970s, Buddhist monks were also main proponents of traditional medicine in the country before the Buddhist *Sangha* was purged in a clamp-down on the independence of monasteries by General Ne Win's BSPP government: see Chapter 5.

[11] Many hospitals in Burma are very small, with sometimes just a dozen beds and one qualified doctor.

[12] *Bangkok Post*, 30 Jan. 1995.

Chapter 4

HEALTH IN A SOCIETY UNDER CENSORSHIP

Burma today has one of the toughest systems of state censorship and media control of any country in the world. The damaging effects of years of censorship and health neglect in Burma are manifold and intrude into every health field. As will be discussed in this chapter, censorship is achieved by both direct means imposed by the authorities, and through the insidious — but equally debilitating — atmosphere of fear that permeates Burmese society and inhibits reporting and discussion of many issues relating to public health. In addition, there is such a paucity of information available on all aspects of public health and health care — and the information that there is often appears sketchy and potentially misleading — that it becomes impossible for informed public debate on policy to develop, and very difficult also for international agencies to plan and implement their humanitarian input in the most effective ways. There is an urgent need for freedom of research and for freedom to disseminate information in this field. Moreover, while certain public emergencies are sporadically addressed through public information campaigns, many of the most common and life-threatening health risks that the Burmese peoples face are not realistically or publicly addressed by the government at all. In its failure to provide readily available information about such risks and how they can be avoided, the Burmese government has for many years demonstrated a negligence that threatens the health — and indeed the lives — of many of its people.

As Burma slowly emerges from the 26-year era of General Ne Win's "Burmese Way to Socialism", a number of changes have occurred in the structure and appearance of the Burmese media, largely in response to economic change. Since 1988, an independent publishing industry that concentrates on business affairs has been allowed to develop, and various new journals occasionally comment on social or health issues. In the past eighteen months, for example, the popular magazines *Thintbawa* and *Kyi-pwa-yay* have both carried articles mentioning AIDS, which were passed by the censors. Any criticism of the authorities or government policy, however, is strictly forbidden under a complex array of draconian censorship laws, and virtually all health education and reporting remains the sole prerogative of the government, which tightly controls all television, radio and daily newspapers.[1]

In the state media, although health is a common topic, no comment is ever permitted which might imply any neglect or failing by the authorities. The state-controlled *New Light of Myanmar*, in particular, often carries news agency reports from international organizations such as the WHO or UNDP, but these are generally concerned with health issues at the global level and do not illustrate actual health conditions in Burma.[2] Instead, local health news consists largely of lists of prominent military, governmental and, on occasion, foreign health figures who have attended various hospital openings, graduation classes or seminars.

Some attempts to address health issues within the country have been obvious propaganda. For example, a recent trilogy of articles in the *New Light of Myanmar* on "Indices of Progress in Myanmar" were studded with graphs showing improvements in the health sector at almost Olympian levels, ostensibly demonstrating "that the takeover by the SLORC was aimed at the common good of the country".[3]

For a reader unfamiliar with Burma, such reports — backed up by the copious use of statistics — can give the impression of an effective system of country-wide response and co-ordination in health care. For example, when plague broke out in India during 1994, the SLORC responded with a high-profile national awareness campaign which was heavily promoted in the state media; guard duty was stepped up at all official entry points from India and attempts were made to control the local rat population.[4]

There should be no doubt, too, that there are many public doctors and health officials who try to react as best they can to any medical emergency within the limitations of the present public system. On 20 May 1995, for example, Dr Mya Than Nwe from the Medical Research Department spoke on state radio about health education after an outbreak of bacterial encephalitis in parts of the Magwe Division and Rakhine State.

However, many local health workers and opposition groups complain that the occasional prominence given to such headline stories can flatter to deceive over the real state of national health provision. Sudden emergencies may be covered, but the majority of ongoing health issues continue unreported and unrecorded in any informative way for Burma's peoples. The problem is further exacerbated by the fact that it is very difficult for local health workers to travel and carry out research under current censorship and security laws, and virtually impossible for them to publicize their findings independently, even when they become aware of serious and unrecognized health problems.

As a result, after over three decades of military rule, the state-controlled press shows little sensitivity to local issues, and for many years has failed to cover health conditions in vast areas of the country, especially in ethnic minority regions where local language publications have been restricted.[5] In recent years UNICEF has produced various health materials, such as *Facts for Life*, in Jinghpaw Kachin, Sgaw Karen, Mon, Shan and several other minority languages, but distribution is limited, and local communities and writers face many obstacles before they can publish any materials themselves. (A number of versions of *Where there is no Doctor,* by Dr David Werner, have also been translated into ethnic minority languages, including Karen and Kachin, but these have mostly been distributed from territories controlled by armed opposition groups.)

At the national level, too, health education is grossly under-resourced and many government staff are unmotivated. As a result, people across the country are ill-informed and have little access to essential information on a broad array of vital issues — from the high incidence of malaria in border regions to such common medical problems as malnutrition, hepatitis, snake-bites, complications arising from backstreet abortions and intestinal illnesses (including both dysentery and cholera). Medical practitioners believe that some health problems, such as malnutrition, are neglected because they are an embarrassment, but others, such as cholera, are politically sensitive to the government because they are deemed to draw the international spotlight to the government's failings. In particular, all countries around the world have faced serious cultural, educational and medical challenges in confronting the issue of HIV/AIDS, but in Burma, despite the obvious spawning ground of local conditions, the health authorities were conspicuously late. By the time the SLORC woke up to the looming scale of the problem, hundreds of thousands of people may already have been infected (see Chapter 7).

In many respects, Burma thus presents a classic case not simply of what the act of censorship deliberately represses or excludes but of how an endemic culture of censorship and restrictions on freedom of expression can prevent vital health issues being explained or even discussed or reported. An obvious but long-standing example of this is the often low take-up rate of public services, even where they have been provided. But, as UN agencies have increasingly found, although traditional beliefs are sometimes responsible, this is frequently due simply to a lack of public education and understanding of what is available.[6]

The resultant lack of both individual and community awareness of many common, but serious, health problems in Burma is often astonishing. Reproductive health, narcotics and HIV/AIDS stand out as areas where successive governments in Burma have failed to ensure that the public is properly informed. The list, however, extends much further. For example, although malaria has long been a major cause of infant mortality, many villagers still believe that they can be infected by such means as eating bananas. The treatment of such global health hazards as tuberculosis, which is re-emerging in Burma, is similarly jeopardized by lack of information and the high drop out rate of sufferers before completing their treatment.[7] Equally striking, international agencies are discovering that attempts to rectify Burma's woefully inadequate sanitation and clean water systems through construction work have proven ineffective without the backup of community participation or health education. As UNICEF recently stated, "Little attention was given to the knowledge, attitudes and practices of beneficiaries."[8]

Another much neglected area of health care is the plight of Burma's large population of disabled people (save for military veterans), whose needs have been perennially under-funded and overlooked. For example, although it has been estimated that anywhere between 3.5 and 5 per cent of the population is blind or in other ways disabled, there are only six specialist schools in the country which can cater in total for a maximum of 400 children.[9] As a result, many parents simply keep blind or disabled children at home. The alternatives are bleak. As one physician remarked, "For many people, to become blind in Burma is virtually to become a beggar."

Of similar concern are the country's many leprosy sufferers. Burma is currently one of the world's six main country centres for leprosy, with over 40,000 registered patients in 1993. Some recent advances have been made in treatment, and an improved multi-drug therapy was introduced into Burma in 1992, once again demonstrating the impact that medical aid, when permitted, can bring. However, the broader health aspects are often neglected, and conditions in many of the "leper villages" vary widely. For example, there were widespread reports of considerable hardship and suffering during the forcible re-location (for reasons unknown to ARTICLE 19) of one leper community near Rangoon to an under-prepared site at Ngasu after the SLORC assumed power. None of these issues, however, is raised or substantively investigated in the state-controlled press.

The lack of national awareness, then, of most of the above health problems can largely be attributed to a combination of poor education, press inertia and apparent governmental indifference. The absence of reporting on many other health problems, however, results from delib-erate censorship.

This is undoubtedly most blatant in the reporting of war and humanitarian issues. For many years, the military government has strictly suppressed all news of casualties as well as reporting of other human rights and humanitarian issues which have a bearing on health, such as forced labour or the treatment of prisoners (see Chapter 6). However, except for human rights abuses, many medical practitioners do not believe that military officers have any obvious reason for sup-pressing health news — except largely one of pride. In this, doctors must also take their share of blame for failing to report problems. As one health official privately explained, "The *Tatmadaw* rules the coun-try just like the Burmese kings. They had a saying: 'Make a big prob-lem a small problem, and make a small problem disappear.' Everyone is fearful of criticism and no one wants to admit mistakes."

Evidence of such fear of failure or criticism can be seen in many quarters today. One example occurred during an outbreak of cholera in several townships in the Rangoon Division in early 1993. Foreign diplomats say the outbreak was never officially publicized and that poster campaigns were discouraged since it was feared they might give international visitors to the country a bad impression of Burma's health situation. Foreign journalists and aid workers, too, often face bureaucratic delays or straight refusals in response to requests to visit certain areas or hospitals. Indeed, at some hospitals foreign visitors have been refused access to the wards; instead, they have to wait for patients to be brought for interview in separate rooms and in the presence of officials. Despite the goodwill of foreign visitors, the authorities, it would appear, are extremely nervous about any negative comments or publicity.

However, perhaps the most contentious area of censorship and misreporting on health issues in Burma is in the publication of official statistics. The apparent readiness of the government to make cavalier use of social statistics was graphically illustrated to the world in 1987 when, in order to be accepted by the UN for Least Developed Country status, the previous national literacy rate of 78.6 per cent (for which Burma had twice won UNESCO prizes in the BSPP era) was dropped to just 18.7 per cent.[10]

Since 1988, the same doubts about the accuracy of government statistics have continued. As one international consultant wrote in a recent report to the UNDP in Burma: "With respect to health, it is hard to evaluate progress because of a lack of reliable data."[11] One of the most controversial statistics is the true figure for military spending as compared to expenditure on education and health. Opposition estimates of over 40 per cent of the national budget being swallowed up by military spending contrast with official government figures which, for many years, have stayed at around 20 per cent. There simply is no access to reliable data to assess such very different claims. But even on the basis of this lower figure, Professor Khin Maung Kyi, a Burmese economist at the National University of Singapore, has demonstrated that, using the criteria employed in the UNDP's Human Development Reports, Burma has the highest military spending as a percentage of government expenditure out of a comparable grouping of regional countries that includes Indonesia, Thailand, Bangladesh and Malaysia — and despite having no external enemies.[12] Equally stark, at around 152 per cent in 1992, Burma had by far the greatest imbalance of military expenditure against health and education spending among these countries, with projections that it could rise to 200 per cent in 1996.[13]

Nonetheless, if many aspects of government and military spending remain shrouded in mystery, there can be little doubt that increasing international scrutiny of Burma's social data in recent years has brought about a new sensitivity over the recycling of questionable information. This has been illustrated in the arguments of Dr Aung Tun Thet, a former Health Ministry official currently working with UNICEF. Dr Thet, for example, has argued that, although by most international political and economic indicators Burma is usually classified with countries "in crisis", such as Afghanistan, Angola, Iraq, Mozambique, Sudan and Zaire, when various health and educational indicators are examined, Burma under the SLORC (or *Nawata*) is actually some way ahead in terms of general social progress.[14] Significantly, Dr Thet also asserts that, although in the past there had been "a tendency to hide the actual situation by producing dubious figures", since 1990 the SLORC has given "explicit directives to ensure the production of accurate social statistics".[15]

Apparent recognition of this need to improve basic health data came with the announcement of the 1993-1996 National Health Plan, when the reliability of national health information was for the first time officially questioned during a workshop by government health workers:

> Monitoring and Evaluation were identified early
> ... as weak spots in the management system ... .
> The participants identified the information from the
> peripheral health units as being incomplete,
> inaccurate, patchy and unreliable for monitoring
> and planning purposes.[16]

Since the publication of the National Health Plan, a number of failings in the health and educational sectors have been discreetly voiced in government reports. For example, the massive educational underachievement of Burma's children and the fact that the majority of children do not complete primary school have been admitted on several occasions. Indeed, the provision of primary health care and universal access to basic education have been publicly heralded as main goals of Burma's National Programme of Action for the Survival, Protection and Development of Myanmar's Children in the 1990s.

Critics of the SLORC, however, allege that government officials, rather than taking necessary actions, are simply becoming more
adept at regurgitating UN development language. Indeed, it is in the
background papers and reports of the UN agencies themselves (notably UNICEF and UNDP) that the underlying health problems are most
explicitly stated. To date, the government has taken few substantive
steps to address most health issues.

For the moment, then, huge doubts must remain over the quality
of basic health information on which current health planning and expenditure are officially based. As with all health statistics in Burma,
there are always wide regional and ethnic disparities which are not
reflected in national figures. Sometimes, even national figures are
changed quite dramatically. The most striking example is the much-
quoted infant mortality rate (IMR), which is widely seen as a main
indicator for national standards of health. In the early 1970s, the IMR
was set by the Health Ministry at around 47 per 1,000 live births (for
children under one), at which level it remained for twenty years,
apparently unchallenged by UNICEF, the WHO and other international
agencies, until 1992 when it was suddenly doubled by the Ministry of
Health to 94 per 1,000 live births. At the same time, the official under-
five mortality rate was similarly doubled to 147 per 1,000 live births,
which is the fourth highest figure amongst the 14 countries in the UN's
East Asia and Pacific Region.

This massive rise in the IMR has been explained by the Central
Statistical Organization of the Ministry of National Planning and Economic Development, which has responsibility for collating all such
social and health data, as reflecting improved statistical methods.
According to this explanation, the earlier rate was incomplete because
it was based largely upon urban statistics, while the new figure is
derived from a broader statistical base. But one public health worker
who was involved in the new survey has privately told ARTICLE 19,
"We could no longer hide the truth." Even more confusingly, while the
new 94 per 1,000 live birth figure is recorded for 1993 in the latest
Health in Myanmar report, a figure of between 47.5 (urban) and 49.6
(rural) is provisionally stated for 1994, suggesting that the authorities
might well be preparing to scale the IMR dramatically downwards
once again.[17]

Not surprisingly, many doctors warn that the reliability of any adjusted figures produced by the government should be treated with great caution. In the case of infant mortality, there are many variations in estimates of the IMR in different localities, which reflect both the paucity of governmental outreach and the very different health conditions in different parts of the country. For example, doctors working with Médecins Sans Frontières (France) have estimated the IMR at around 200 per 1,000 live births in war-torn ethnic Karen regions along the Thai-Burma border while, by some estimates, the figure in upland areas of the eastern Shan State could be as high as 300 per 1,000 live births.[18] Towards the other end of the scale, and despite the many local health problems, in some of the new towns around Rangoon health workers have calculated the IMR in these areas as being below the 1993 national average — at closer to 65 per 1,000 live births.

Finally, it needs to be stressed that simple concentration on data collection and the reliability of statistics can be very misleading in judging the overall state of health emergency, provision and delivery in Burma. After recent tours of the country, a number of international health and development workers have privately said that in some areas the health infrastructures are either non-existent or so poor that official statistics simply cannot reflect the real conditions of health in the community. In many rural areas, for example, cholera and dysentery epidemics, which take hundreds of lives, still go unreported or uninvestigated inside Burma, especially in ethnic minority areas and the war zones.[19] Explained one foreign aid official, who asked to remain anonymous:

> It's all very well for health officials to use statistical projections to declare a state of emergency over the spread of AIDS — and they may well be right. But for many families and communities it will still be malaria, conflict or malnutrition and poverty brought on by everyday social injustices and hardship that will continue to take the greatest toll of life. However there is no sense of governmental or international urgency over issues like these.

Indeed, many local health workers already feel that the tendency of international donor agencies to focus on the high-profile issue of HIV/AIDS could help to marginalize vulnerable groups and other long-standing health problems even further. "Nowadays people will train in AIDS but nobody wants to work in a leper colony or work with the blind or handicapped," one physician complained. "Doctors will only work where they know there are good salaries and funds."

Another concern expressed about official statistics is that they do not reflect the quality of health care that is actually provided. One veteran official in the Burmese health system privately made a long list of criticisms:

> The way health statistics have been used in official reports is unethical and misleading. The survey questions asked to produce such data never reveal the true picture. There is no proper monitoring or feed-back. For example, there is always a lot of statistical concentration or publicity about the opening of new clinics or hospitals, but it is never asked or disclosed whether there has been a better rate of diagnosis, more doctors employed or patients seen, a better rate of treatment, a better rate of patient satisfaction or an improvement in the general standards of health in the community. This is what we should be aiming at, but no one dares openly talk or write about it.

A similarly neglected issue is the manner in which the central government in Burma has been able to use its control over both health provision and the media for its own political purposes. This is a trend which has accelerated under the SLORC. For example, after decades of neglect in most ethnic minority regions, the SLORC has been publicly offering the sudden prospect of hospitals, doctors, and access to foreign aid agencies and medical supplies in areas where the military authorities have an agenda for change; other minority areas, however, remain neglected. The one message constantly reinforced in the state media is that the military government is the only institution in the country which can provide such beneficial developments and which, by implication, should be the only conduit for international aid and funds. Opposition groups, on the other hand, believe that the provision of aid solely through government channels is more likely to empower the SLORC than the people it is intended to help. In achieving health solutions, all sectors — both governmental and non-governmental — must ultimately be expected to play a role. But, for the moment, there remain vast areas of the country where international aid workers have no access to the community to judge the health realities or social infrastructures for themselves.

Finally, perhaps the most overlooked area of censorship and health care are the health rights of the Burmese peoples themselves, especially the right to information. In a health system where corruption is widespread and private practice booming, many people have increasingly fallen victim to a pernicious combination of press control and exploitation by unscrupulous doctors who do not hesitate to conceal information as well. Explained one physician:

> The problem is often not so much one of censorship in itself, but a complete lack of information or fora for citizens to discuss health issues which they need to know about in their daily lives. This means that they are totally vulnerable, not only to preventable illnesses or diseases such as malaria, HIV or cholera, but also to doctors in whom they put their trust. Many doctors will always direct them in the direction of the private sector where they can make lots of money through treatments and drugs. The patients, however, are unable to judge the diagnosis, context or quality of any treatment they receive.

Although there are many incidents of individual generosity by doctors, misdiagnosis and poor treatment are common. Equally serious is the uncontrolled sale and mishandling of medicines by both doctors and middlemen who make their living out of this trade. The country's National Drug Law has never been strictly enforced. In fact, the state-owned Burma Pharmaceutical Industry (BPI) is one of the few governmental institutions that has historically enjoyed a high reputation for quality in the country, but production is generally limited and most medicines are always in short supply. As a result, in the days of the BSPP a thriving cross-border trade in black market medicines developed, which was estimated to account for over 50 per cent of all drugs on sale in the country.[20]

Under the SLORC's market-oriented economic system, parts of the border trade have become technically legal. However, problems in both commercial distribution and sales persist with exactly the same negative implications for patients. No health regulations are visibly employed to govern the prescription or labelling of medicines. On sale in the markets are many fake products and out-of-date medicines, as well as drugs bearing instructions in only Chinese, Thai or Indian languages, which few medical practitioners — let alone ordinary inhabitants — can read. Contraceptive pills, for example, are often sold in loose strips, devoid of any instructions or packaging. Moreover such unsound medical practices are not only confined to the private sector, which accounts for the bulk of this trade. One confidential survey in a public health centre recently monitored dispensing practices according to WHO standards and found them "far from rational"; indeed, none of the medicines at the clinic were labelled with prescription instructions at all.

The discovery of such malpractice can place international agencies in a difficult moral dilemma. In a system where little objective or investigative reporting has ever been allowed, foreign organizations can be quickly seen as troublemakers if they publicize their findings, causing embarrassment or arousing resentment among government officials and local doctors alike. As a result, the need for publicity to spread awareness is often tempered by self-censorship and tact in order to be allowed to continue working and to try and produce long-term results.

One issue, however, on which public information campaigns are urgently needed concerns the dangers of intravenous treatments carried out in unhygienic conditions, particularly in a context of rising HIV-infection. Initially introduced by doctors as another means of selling more medicines, intravenous treatments, especially drips and vitamin injections, are extremely popular. Chinese-brand injections, especially B-Complex or B-12-1,000, are commonplace and are desired by patients as a means of boosting energy levels during illness. Standards of hygiene, however, leave a lot to be desired in even public health centres where new or sterilized needles are always in short supply, but the fashion for giving vitamin injections is also endemic amongst the many unregistered practitioners working throughout the country.

In the Kachin State, for example, quacks — who use unsterilized needles — claim to provide three years' protection against malaria by injection. What is actually in these injections has not been surveyed (some reportedly contain opium or heroin). But many of those who seek such backstreet treatments are heroin addicts, amongst whom alarmingly high rates of HIV-infection are now being detected (see Chapter 7).

Like many health issues in Burma, state restrictions and negligence mean that the scale of this problem has yet to be properly researched. It could be a local problem that is tied to the lifestyle and culture of intravenous drug users in north-east Burma. Some medical experts, however, are not so sure. They believe that many people may have already been unwittingly infected. "A time bomb" was the private verdict of one government doctor.

NOTES

[1] See, ARTICLE 19, *State of Fear*, and ARTICLE 19, *Censorship Prevails* (see Chapter 1, note 4). Despite being allowed to write on some social topics, the January 1996 issue of *Thintbawa* had over 50 out of 160 pages on the subject of education in Burma torn out by the censors.

[2] See e.g., *New Light of Myanmar*, 19 Nov. 1993, for an article taken from *World Health* (magazine of the World Health Organization) on the global fight against tuberculosis.

[3] *New Light of Myanmar*, 29, 30 and 31 Aug. 1995. According to the paper, this report was prepared for the American oil company, UNOCAL, by a consultancy firm, International Security Management, Inc.

[4] Ibid., 2 Oct. 1994. Though little publicized, there are still occasional outbreaks of plague — usually the bubonic form — in the central dry zone region of Burma. A Health Ministry official privately admitted 528 cases and three deaths in one such epidemic in 1992.

[5] ARTICLE 19, *Censorship Prevails,* note 1 above, at 35-38.

[6] UNICEF, *Children and Women in Myanmar* (see Chapter 2, note 13), 51.

[7] In one recent, unpublished survey of tuberculosis patients in an urban community, less than 10 per cent finished one year of treatment and, of these, three-quarters had dropped out within four months.

[8] UNICEF, *Children and Women in Myanmar,* note 6 above, at 61. There are still many communities in Burma where the importance of clean water is not understood, and where untreated water from rivers or shallow wells is sometimes preferred to water from deep tube-wells and boiled water.

[9] Ibid., at 65.

[10] ARTICLE 19, *State of Fear,* note 1 above, at 27. The true figure is probably closer to 70 per cent (with considerable variation in different ethnic regions), and it is this higher estimate that most international agencies use today. A particular problem in establishing reliable figures is assessing the quality of literacy taught in Buddhist monasteries which, in the absence of other schools, have often been the main source of learning for rural villagers.

[11] Dr D Dapice, *Prospects for Sustainable Growth in Myanmar/Burma: Tensions between environmental decline and economic progress: A Report to the United Nations Development Programme* (Harvard Institute for International Development, 12 Sept. 1995), 6.

[12] Prof. Khin Maung Kyi, *Burmese Gleam: Will it Endure and Glow or Flicker and Die? A Prognosis of Recent Economic Changes in Burma* (discussion paper, Washington: Oct. 1995), 10-11.

[13] Ibid.

[14] Dr A T Thet, *"Nawata's* Performance in the Social Sectors: The Untold Story"* (conference paper, Burma Studies Colloquium, North Illinois University: Oct. 1994), 1.

[15] Ibid., at 8.

[16] Ministry of Health, *Union of Myanmar: National Health Plan* (see Chapter 3, note 3), 10.

[17] Ministry of Health, *Health in Myanmar 1996* (Rangoon: 1996), 81-82.

[18] D Porter, *Wheeling and Dealing: HIV/AIDS and Development on the Shan State Borders* (Background paper supported by UNDP, Rangoon Institute of Economics and Australian National University, Oct. 1994), 29.

[19] For example, in 1993, after several hundred villagers suddenly died in a number of localities in south-eastern Burma due to symptoms that included severe diarrhoea, rumours became rife that the *Tatmadaw* was using biologi-

cal weapons dropped from the air. Samples were smuggled out by Western journalists for testing by British defence experts at Porton Down, but the results were inconclusive. The SLORC has always denied the allegations. Some analysts, by contrast, believe that a more plausible explanation is the recent spread of a new strain of cholera, known as *Vibrio cholerae* 0139 or "Bengal" cholera, which is extremely virulent. For a discussion, see, A Selth, *Transforming the Tatmadaw: The Burmese Armed Forces since 1988* (Canberra Papers on Strategy and Defence No.113, Australian National University: 1996), 120-124.

[20] In the 1980s, the BPI share of the market was estimated at around 25 per cent, other drug imports by the government at 17 per cent, and medicines distributed by UNICEF or other foreign aid agencies at 4-5 per cent; see, M Roemer, *Primary Health Care in Burma's National Health System* (Rangoon: USAID, 1986), 52.

Chapter 5

POLITICAL RESTRICTIONS ON MEDICAL PRACTITIONERS

Doctors and other health workers have traditionally formed one of the most respected sectors in Burmese society. Doctors, however, who have participated in opposition political activities, or who have spoken out against the government, are among those whom the security services have particularly targeted for repression. In addition, the medical profession as a whole suffers from the severe restrictions on freedom of expression and association that also apply to other occupational groups in Burma.

In the parliamentary era of the 1950s, although there were many failings within the national health system, hospitals and physicians in Burma enjoyed international renown. The door remained open to the international community, and many ethnic Indians continued to work as doctors in both the private and public sectors. Foreign diplomats and other patients, for example, would often travel from Thailand and other neighbouring countries for specialist treatment in Rangoon.

Medical practitioners date the general decline in specialist standards to the military's seizure of power in 1962 and the beginning of 26 years of isolation under General Ne Win's *Burmese Way to Socialism*. As political repression mounted, all industries were nationalized and most foreigners expelled, prompting a steady exodus of qualified doctors which has continued until today. Currently, several thousand doctors from Burma are believed to be working abroad.

Most emigrant Burmese doctors admit to having left for either financial or political reasons which, until recently, strictly precluded their return.[1] However, many also felt frustrated by the fall in medical training standards that followed the nationalization of all schools and colleges in 1964. In particular, the abolition of the Chair of English at Rangoon University in 1966 and the demotion of English to a minor subject in schools proved a serious handicap to medical students. With funds always scarce, translations of scientific texts never kept pace with demand, and the publication of essential training materials was further delayed by bureaucracy and censorship.

Finally, this damaging discrimination against English was ended in 1980 after one of General Ne Win's own daughters was rumoured to have failed entrance tests to begin postgraduate studies in medicine abroad. The damage, however, had already been done to a whole generation of students. Although some excellent medical staff have remained in the country, there is a general consensus that educational standards have never recovered. Certainly, insufficient doctors or nurses were trained to staff the expansion in health care that was attempted under the BSPP. On paper, many of the Health Ministry's goals looked sound but, other than increased immunization, few targets were successfully reached due to a combination of ill-conceived policies and the continuing state of political crisis in the country.

Since 1988, the social and political pressures on medical practitioners have greatly intensified, as they have for all other public servants. Young doctors and medical students were highly active in the democracy protests of 1988. A number of undergraduates from Rangoon Institute of Medicine No.2, for example, were in the line of fire when troops began shooting at demonstrators outside the United States' Embassy on 19 September, the day after the SLORC assumed power. Eyewitnesses said that, elsewhere in the city, nurses and medical personnel, including one carrying a Red Cross flag, were shot at by the security forces when they went to try and help some of the wounded.[2] In the aftermath of these shootings, a number of well-known doctors and medical students joined the several thousand democracy activists who fled into territory controlled by armed ethnic opposition groups following the SLORC's assumption of power. Prominent among them were Dr Naing Aung and Dr Thaung Htun, both leading figures in the All Burma Students Democratic Front (ABSDF), which is still militarily active and runs health programmes of its own in a few border regions today.

In government-controlled areas, meanwhile, the political pressures on medical practitioners have been relentless. Like all universities and colleges of higher education, Burma's four main institutes of medicine were periodically closed by the authorities for much of 1988-1991. Even though medical classes resumed before other faculties, another massive backlog in the training and qualification of health personnel was caused. By early 1991, huge staffing gaps were appearing in many of the country's hospitals and clinics. Then, in another intensification of pressure on public servants, in April 1991 all doctors employed in the public sector — like other civil servants — were barred from engaging in politics under SLORC decree No.1/91 and required to fill in forms answering 33 detailed questions on their political views, including about the *Tatmadaw*, insurgent groups, the NLD leader Aung San Suu Kyi, the US Central Intelligence Agency and the British Broadcasting Corporation (BBC). Subsequently, hundreds more medical personnel were reported to have been sacked on the basis of their answers, bringing to 15,000 the number of civil servants that Lieutenant-General Khin Nyunt announced had been sacked or disciplined since the SLORC came to power.[3]

However, perhaps the most extraordinary crack-down on doctors and other public health workers occurred the following year. Following student demonstrations at Rangoon University in December 1991 in celebration of the award of the Nobel Peace Prize to Aung San Suu Kyi, in early 1992 the SLORC ordered all government doctors to attend "re-education" courses run by the Military Intelligence Service at the former BSPP training camp at Phaungyii, where civil servants had also been made to attend political training classes under the previous government. Nearly 3,000 — a quarter of the country's doctors — attended the first six courses during 1992-1993. Dressed in military uniforms, they were required to attend classes aimed at providing "doctors with nationalism", "acceptance" of the military's leading role, "management of public health affairs" and the "observance of discipline".[4] Yet again, the political behaviour and attitudes of health workers were closely monitored and, following the completion of these courses, colleagues reported that a number of doctors and other health officials were abruptly dismissed.

After seven years of such constant scrutiny and political observation, many doctors say that the triple pressures of political censorship and poor working conditions and low wages have left even the most committed of the country's public health workers a very demoralized force. As in other walks of civil service life, a common saying among health workers runs: "Ma loke — Ma shoke — Ma pyoke: no work — no problems — no sackings." Moreover, while there is no evidence that doctors have been prevented from carrying out their daily medical work, there is a deep-felt view that, like other intellectuals, writers and academics, they are especially vulnerable to being targeted by the government because of their social status and potential influence should they dare to express dissent. Explained one doctor, "It's OK as long as you just do your job and keep away from politics. But if you are a doctor and do get involved, then you are in immediate danger."

There is considerable evidence to support such claims. Doctors have been prominent amongst opposition figures arrested or imprisoned by the SLORC since 1988. Dr Zaw Min, for example, who participated in the 1988 protests at Rangoon University and Rangoon General Hospital, was arrested in July 1989 and subsequently sentenced to 20 years' imprisonment with hard labour (since reduced to 10) under section 5(j) of the 1950 Emergency Provisions Act for allegedly distributing seditious anti-government literature and illegally organizing workers. Like another physician who was also arrested, Dr Maw Zin from Paukkhaung, he was suspected of involvement with the outlawed Communist Party of Burma.

The main security pressures, however, have been focused on medical supporters of the National League for Democracy. In an apparent act of revenge, Dr Tin Myo Win, an NLD central committee member and surgeon at Rangoon General Hospital, was arrested in August 1989 on vague security charges for what many fellow professionals believe was his active support for the 1988 democracy movement. Dr Win was eventually released in 1992 but many more NLD supporters, including several well-known medical figures, have continued to be arrested and imprisoned. On 30 April 1991, for example, two respected physicians, Dr Zaw Myint Maung, the elected Member of Parliament (MP) for Amarapura-1, and Dr Zaw Myint, MP-elect for Henzada-2, were both sentenced to 25 years' imprisonment on imprecise sedition charges for allegedly planning to "set up an illegal government".[5] In March 1996, Dr Zaw Myint also received an additional 12 year sentence under the Penal Code and section 5(j) of the Emergency Provisions Act as part of a group of 21 political prisoners in Insein jail who were convicted of offences likely to "disrupt" the morality, security or stability of the country. The evidence offered against them was the possession of alleged anti-government materials, including a letter describing poor health conditions in the prison, which had been smuggled out to the UN Special Rapporteur to Myanmar (see Chapter 6.3).

In another clamp-down in October 1993, two more well-known medical figures, Dr Aung Khin Sint, also an NLD MP-elect and medical writer, and Dr Ma Thida, a writer and surgeon at the Muslim Free Hospital in Rangoon, were both sentenced to 20 years' imprisonment after being convicted on a variety of charges, including under the 1950 Emergency Provisions Act, the 1962 Printers and Publishers Registration Law and the 1908 Unlawful Associations Act, for allegedly writing "illegal" literature in support of the NLD and distributing it during the SLORC's National Convention in Rangoon.[6] After months of pressure by the UN Special Rapporteur to Myanmar, Dr Aung Khin Sint was unexpectedly released in February 1995, but Dr Ma Thida, who has reportedly suffered from tuberculosis, remains in prison amid growing concerns about her health (see Chapter 6.3).

However, perhaps the clearest evidence of the political harassment of a medical practitioner has been the experience of Dr Khin Zaw Win (also known as Kelvin). A qualified dentist and former UNICEF worker, Khin Zaw Win attended the UN Conference on the Rights of the Child in China in 1992. Subsequently, he embarked on a postgraduate degree programme at the University of Singapore and continued his contact with international health officials. Briefly back in Burma, he was arrested at Mingaladon Airport on 4 July 1994 and later sentenced to 15 years' imprisonment for allegedly "spreading false news" and other offences. In a broad array of charges, he was convicted under the 1950 Emergency Provisions Act (5e), Section 17/1 of the Unlawful Associations Act and Section 5 of the 1923 Official Secrets Act as well as on various currency and customs charges. Colleagues, however, believe that the latter charges were merely intended as an attempt to discredit him. The real reason for his arrest, they say, was his academic research into Burmese politics and his well-known contacts with foreigners, including the UN's Special Rapporteur to Myanmar to whom the *New Light of Myanmar* alleged he had helped send "fabricated news" in 1992.[7]

Khin Zaw Win's only "offence", it thus appears, was that he had tried to speak out. In a conference paper distributed in Australia, he had written in poignant terms of the consequences of political deadlock and the need for peaceful reform:

> Understandably, there are now signs of ideological
> fatigue, a vacuum so to speak. The censorship that
> has prevailed at all levels during the last three dec-
> ades has been terribly effective.[8]

The use of such smear charges against prominent individuals accused
of expressing anti-government opinions is not unusual. The most striking example also occurred in the medical field, in 1989, when U Win
Tin, vice-chairman of Burma's Writers Association and a central
committee member of the NLD, was arrested on trumped up charges
of being involved in an illegal abortion. His link to the case was
tenuous; a young man whose partner had recently undergone an abortion briefly stayed at his house. Nevertheless, in October 1989 he and
another NLD colleague, U Ngwe Hlaing, were sentenced under
section 216 of the Penal Code to three years' hard labour for allegedly
"harbouring an offender".[9] Abortion is illegal in Burma, but prosecu-
tions are rarely brought. However, while the young couple and doctor
who carried out the abortion have since been released, Win Tin was
kept in jail after reportedly receiving a further 11 year sentence under
the 1950 Emergency Provisions Act for reasons that have never been
publicly disclosed. In March 1996, Win Tin also received an additional five year sentence along with Dr Zaw Myint and 19 other
prisoners who had been accused of anti-government activities in jail,
including writing to the UN Special Rapporteur to Myanmar (see Chapter 6.3). Now 65 years old, Win Tin is in poor health after over six
years without adequate medical treatment and is suffering from chronic
spondylitis, for which he has to wear a neck brace.

Finally, in addition to the repression suffered by individual doctors and medical practitioners who participate in opposition politics,
the profession as a whole suffers severe restrictions on its right to
organize and the right to freedom of association. Independent trade
union activity, which had briefly revived during the 1988 protests,
was immediately banned following the SLORC's assumption of power.
Instead, health workers who want to involve themselves in voluntary
medical associations are largely restricted to three organizations, all
of which — although described as "NGOs" — have close links to the
Health Ministry and government. This creates particular problems for

foreign NGOs and UN agencies working in Burma, which are increasingly being required, in response to international concern, to try to work with independent and representative NGOs in the community. Yet, it is these very government-backed NGOs, as well as the Health Ministry and local township authorities, which the SLORC has been urging international organizations to accept as local partners.

After years of political repression and malaise, the question of indigenous NGOs in Burma is a difficult one. In fact, independent NGOs of the kind envisaged by international agencies have never become fully established. For a variety of political and cultural reasons, despite the traditional generosity of the Burmese peoples towards community projects, indigenous NGOs dealing with local or specialist issues (such as disabilities, drug addiction or ethnic nationality questions) have either been prohibited or never properly developed — and this has long applied in armed opposition territory as well as in government-controlled areas.

Founded in 1949, Burma's oldest NGO, the Myanmar Medical Association (MMA), began life as a professional association and currently has over 6,000 members, with 50 branches at the township or state/divisional levels. Consisting of physicians from both the public and private sectors, the MMA was pulled into the government's orbit during the time of the BSPP when senior officials in the Ministry of Health took up key leadership posts in its governing hierarchy. However, although the MMA continues to publish its own journal and run occasional workshops and programmes (including an AIDS prevention project with World Vision in Kawthaung), many health workers feel that the MMA has yet to re-establish its independence under the present SLORC government.

This has largely left the non-governmental health field to Burma's two other main "NGOs", the Myanmar Red Cross (MRC) and the Myanmar Maternal and Child Welfare Association (MMCWA), both of which have even closer links with the government and Ministry of Health. With over 180,000 volunteer members, the MRC is supported by public donations and government funds and is supposed to have branches in each of the country's 319 townships. Here its primary role is disaster preparedness and first aid to complement public services. Similarly, the MMCWA is also trying to establish branches in townships throughout the country. As it expands, one of its main tasks will be to work with local Township Medical Officers, under the Ministry of Health, to manage many of the country's Maternal and Child Health Centres.

That there are many committed doctors and health workers in both organizations is not in question. Doubts, however, have been frequently raised over the neutrality and responsibilities of these organizations in the current political environment. For example, in over four decades of armed conflict, there is no evidence of the MRC ever operating as a neutral, humanitarian agency among civilian communities in armed opposition areas. By contrast, in 1989 the MRC became involved in the controversial repatriation of several hundred student refugees from Thailand and more recently, in 1994-1995, in the repatriation of over 190,000 Muslim refugees from Bangladesh, when victims of human rights abuses were allegedly sent back against their will to Burma (see Chapter 6.2). Indeed, opposition groups allege that Military Intelligence officers and informers are routinely placed within the MRC's ranks, causing many communities — especially ethnic minorities — to view the MRC as another branch of government.

Likewise, even the treatment of children is not free from political argument, and the MMCWA's NGO status is also often questioned. Its joint General-Secretary (a doctor) is the wife of the SLORC Secretary-One, Lieutenant-General Khin Nyunt; the President is the wife of Colonel Pe Thein, the former health minister; and the Vice-President is the sister of the late Dr Maung Maung, a leading BSPP functionary and, originally, one of Ne Win's chosen successors as party chairman.

Equally critical, at a time of historic social and economic change, many people believe that the obvious favouritism shown by the SLORC towards the MMA, MRC and MMCWA is inhibiting the development of other independent NGOs, which could more accurately reflect the aspirations of the different ethnic peoples of Burma. Experience the world over has demonstrated that the existence of such popular and democratic institutions is fundamental to the building of civil society and integral to sustainable development and political reform.

In response to such concerns by donor governments, in 1992 the UNDP's Governing Council decided to reorientate its programmes in Burma towards the grass roots level.[10] Since this time, as the door to Burma slowly opens, a number of foreign NGOs and UN agencies have been urging the Burmese health authorities to accept that effective health care is based upon genuine participation by local communities. This important ideal, however, would appear contradicted by events inside Burma. For not only has the SLORC continued to reject the democratic aspirations of the Burmese peoples, as expressed in the result of the 1990 general election, but any members of society, who are suspected of anti-government opinions, face discrimination in gaining public positions or forming or joining local organizations of their choice. In many townships, for example, NLD supporters have been barred from school parents' and teachers' associations. Opposition groups thus claim that the provision of all aid is still politically dominated by the SLORC-led government.

In the ethnic minority war zones, too, the issue of NGOs and community participation is equally controversial. Here, central government outreach has long been resisted; but, in agreeing to cease-fires, many armed opposition groups have told their supporters that economic development, the legalization of indigenous NGOs, and the construction of a new system of public health care are all activities which can help cement the peace. Yet, the SLORC has been reluctant to authorize any new projects in which locally-based community or opposition groups are actively involved. Instead, international aid agencies are required to negotiate first with the SLORC and relevant government ministries over access at the community level. To date, no major development project has been begun under ethnic minority auspices.

The result is widespread dissatisfaction with the quality and level of access to health care that has been provided so far. The reality falls far short of the image of new building programmes for health which are constantly projected in the state-controlled media. The SLORC, for example, claimed to have constructed over 30 hospitals and 66 dispensaries under its Border Areas Development Programme between 1989 and 1993 alone.[11] However, Kyauk Nyi Lai, Secretary-General of the United Wa State Party, which signed a cease-fire with the SLORC as long ago as 1989, has provided a markedly different picture:

> The SLORC claims it helps the Wa but, for example, when it builds a hospital, there is neither a bed nor a single doctor. And when I ask the Burmese

why they do that, they answer "we have our own problems".[12]

Fundamental problems, therefore, lie ahead concerning the rights to freedom of association, participation and expression if local communities and groups in Burma are to be allowed to take control of their own health destinies. Many community groups and leaders are willing to accept this important task. In addition to opposition political groups, many community or religious-based groups — including Buddhist, Christian and Muslim organizations — are keen to expand the scope of their activities to help meet the needs of their communities. Over the years, for example, several Christian-based groups have been permitted to undertake educational projects in fields as diverse as AIDS awareness to running kindergarten classes. In addition to the Christian churches, Muslim or Buddhist organizations, such as the Young Men's Buddhist Association, also run orphanages, and in some areas Buddhist monks, who were once the country's main suppliers of traditional medicine, have recently begun to expand their role in working with local drug addicts or AIDS-sufferers. Under existing legislation, however, religious organizations are barred from straying outside a strictly religious mandate. Existing programmes remain technically under evangelical auspices: and one of the reasons why the former BSPP government moved to purge the Buddhist *Sangha* in the late 1970s was to prevent the country's estimated 150,000 monks from playing such a social role, which was deemed to bring them into possible opposition or competition with the authorities. Indeed, political pressures on Buddhist organizations, in particular, have intensified under the SLORC.[13] Furthermore, despite the obvious popularity of such religious-based organizations within their communities, the SLORC still appears undecided if it will allow any of these groups — whether Buddhist, Christian or Muslim — to become local partners to international aid organizations in any large-scale or significant way.[14]

For the present, then, it is only the MMA, MRC and MMCWA, all of which maintain national structures, which are the main NGOs able to function in the health field. To try and address this issue, in January 1996 the NLD unveiled a development strategy whereby international agencies, such as the UNDP, should work with the NLD

as the only national organization in Burma that had been democrati-
cally shown to represent the will of the people. The party welcomed,
NLD leaders said, the creation and work of indigenous NGOs in the
community. In this way, by following the primary objectives of the
UNDP's Human Development Initiative[15], the NLD considered that
humanitarian and development aid could be more ethically targeted
by democracy supporters at the poorest and most disadvantaged members of society.

To support this new policy, Aung San Suu Kyi, General-
Secretary of the NLD, attempted to institute an official dialogue —
both through correspondence and face-to-face meetings — with leaders of different UN agencies responsible for development and health.
This prompted a furious reaction from the SLORC. After Suu Kyi met
in February 1996 with Giorgio Giacomelli, Executive Director of the
UN International Drug Control Programme (UNDCP), the state-
controlled *New Light of Myanmar* accused him of conduct "incompat-
ible with the status of a gentleman" and made a racist slur against the
British husband of Suu Kyi:

> While in Myanmar, Mr Giorgio Giacomelli was
> treated well. But under the arrangement of the
> UNDP Resident Representative, he stealthily met
> the wife of the man with the long nose at the UNDP
> office in the afternoon of 11 February 96. He did
> so in disregard of the hospitality extended to him,
> without paying attention to his dignity and not in
> concert with his job. He then had clandestine dis-
> cussions not in favour of drug control measures
> taken in Myanmar.[16]

Shortly afterwards, a flight carrying the head of the World Health Organization, was reportedly delayed without explanation for two hours
in Mandalay to prevent him returning to Rangoon in time for a scheduled meeting with Suu Kyi.

The SLORC thus appears determined to monopolize or control
all contacts between international agencies and representatives of the
peoples of Burma. In contrast to the work of the NLD and other
indigenous groups in the community, many doctors in Burma believe

that the next organization to receive the same preferential treatment as the MRC and MMCWA will be the government-backed Union Solidarity and Development Association (USDA), a mass organization formed in late 1993 after the SLORC's earlier attempt to form a successor party to the BSPP failed to gain popular support. With an estimated two million members, the USDA is now organized by the authorities throughout most SLORC-controlled areas of the country and frequently mobilized, in mass rallies, to demonstrate community backing for all the government's plans. Despite its quasi-political status, in early 1996 the USDA was included in a list of "national NGOs" approved by the Health Ministry.[17] Indeed, international health workers report that USDA representatives already sit in, as a matter of course, on planning meetings and health seminars in many townships. In Sittwe, for example, the Rakhine State capital, the MMCWA is even located in the USDA building.

NOTES

[1] The 1982 Citizenship Law barred citizens who had left Burma and taken foreign citizenship from returning. Since the lifting of this ban in 1993, increasing numbers of exiled doctors have revisited their country, although it is not certain whether any have re-established residence.

[2] See e.g., Physicians for Human Rights, *Health and Human Rights in Burma (Myanmar)* (Boston: 1991), 8-9; and *Burma: Dying for Democracy* (Channel Four TV, UK, 15 March 1989).

[3] Rangoon Home Service, 4 Oct. 1991; ARTICLE 19, *State of Fear* (see Chapter 1, note 4), 61-62. Doctors also complain that, where more than one family member is working in public service, another form of punishment is the compulsory transfer of husbands, wives or other close relatives to different regions of the country.

[4] *New Light of Myanmar*, 27 May 1993.

[5] Dr Myint Naing, NLD MP-elect for Kanbalu-2, also received a 25 year prison term after his arrest in October 1990, but his trial details have not been reported.

[6] For trial details, see, ARTICLE 19, *Censorship Prevails* (see Chapter 1, note 4), 8-9 and 28.

[7] *New Light of Myanmar*, 23 Aug. 1994.

[8] Dr Khin Zaw Win, *The State, Order and Prospects for Change in Burma* (Conference paper distributed at The Centre for the Study of Australia-Asia Relations, Griffith University, 3-4 Dec. 1992), 2.

[9] Amnesty International, *Myanmar (Burma): Prisoners of Conscience: A Chronicle of Events since September 1988* (London: 1989), 56-57.

[10] UNDP, *Summary Report: UNDP Assistance to Myanmar*. See Chapter 2, note 19.

[11] Ministry of the Development of Border Areas and National Races, *Measures Taken for Development of Border Areas and National Races (4)* (Rangoon: 1993), 45-46.

[12] *The Sunday Post* (Bangkok), 2 April 1995.

[13] See, ARTICLE 19, *State of Fear,* note 3 above, at 62-66. For example, after monks organized a boycott of religious services for military personnel and their families in protest at the SLORC's refusal to recognize the 1990 general election result, over 350 monasteries were raided by the security services and hundreds of monks detained in October 1990. Then, on 31 October 1990, a new "Law Relating to the *Sangha* Organization" was declared by the SLORC, decreeing that there should be only one Buddhist organization in Burma with nine legally-approved sects.

[14] In 1996, the Christian-based Myanmar Council of Churches was the only religious NGO in Burma on the Health Ministry's list; see note 17 below.

[15] For an analysis of such UNDP operations, see, *UNDP'S Myanmar Human Development Initiative: An Assessment*, prepared for UNDP by Agrodev Canada Inc. (Ontario, January 1995). NLD supporters, however, have questioned a lack of documentary evidence in the report to support its generally positive conclusions.

[16] *New Light of Myanmar*, 22 Feb. 1996.

[17] In addition to the MMCWA, MRC and MMA, the other "NGOs" were the Myanmar "Dental", "Nurses" and "Health Assistant" Associations, all of which are very small, as well as the Myanmar Council of Churches, the only NGO — other than the USDA — to have a non-medical/professional social base; see, Ministry of Health, *Health in Myanmar 1996* (see Chapter 4, note 17), 60.

Chapter 6

CONFLICT AND HUMANITARIAN CRISIS

B urma today is confronted by a host of complex humanitarian issues related to both health and human rights. Many are long-standing problems dating back to Burma's independence in 1948. However, for present-day purposes, they largely fall into three broad categories: death and other physical sufferings resulting from the conduct of war; refugee protection and the internal displacement of civilians; and, finally, the welfare and treatment of prisoners and detainees. All these issues have grave health implications, and have long been veiled under a cloak of censorship which has precluded the development of desperately needed solutions.

6.1 The Backdrop Of War

Undoubtedly the most neglected area of health care in Burma is the humanitarian crisis that exists in many rural areas as a result of over four decades of armed conflict. Virtually all areas of the country have been affected at some stage. There are communities in the Delta and Pegu Yoma regions of Lower Burma, for example, that still suffer from impoverishment and malnutrition as a result of displacement during fighting over 20 years ago. Since the late 1970s, however, the crisis has been most deeply felt in Burma's ethnic minority borderlands, where the human and economic cost of war has been devastating. Ethnic minority peoples constitute an estimated third of the 46 million population and, even today, there are over 20 different ethnic nationalist forces still under arms — both with or without cease-fires with the government.

Until 1988, civilian casualties and the state of civil war in Burma were scarcely mentioned in the state-controlled press. When armed opposition groups were referred to, they were usually described as "bandits", "opium smugglers" or "racist saboteurs". The one exception was on Armed Forces Day in March each year when the government would usually acknowledge the deaths of several hundred troops in the preceding twelve months as opposed to an average 2,500 "insurgents". Opposition forces, by contrast, have estimated the death rate — including civilian victims — at around 10,000 each year, with large annual fluctuations depending on the intensity of the fighting.[1] Certainly, the documented casualty rates among several ethnic minority groups have been appalling. In north-east Burma, for example, the Kachin Independence Organization recorded the deaths of 33,336 civilians in the years 1961-1986 alone, while an unpublished UN survey undertaken in 1991 in Tachilek district in the Shan State revealed a ratio of 1,430 females to 1,000 males, indicating a high mortality rate for ethnic minority men in the fighting.[2]

Such estimates, however, do not give an adequate picture of the degree of human suffering. In ethnic minority areas, in particular, many local communities and cultures have been badly afflicted, and across the country there are countless disabled, widowed or orphaned children among all ethnic groups. Moreover, while General Ne Win's xenophobic *Burmese Way to Socialism* held sway, no independent monitoring of the humanitarian situation was permitted at all within Burma. Neutral observers, including the International Committee of the Red Cross, were strictly barred from the war zones, and no reference was ever made to such important international protocols as the 1949 Geneva Conventions on the Protection of the Victims of War, which set universal minimum standards of humanitarian protection during times of war.[3]

As a result, a systematic pattern of human rights abuses and breaches of international humanitarian law has developed in Burma, in which the summary arrest, torture or extrajudicial execution of civilians have become commonplace, and humane treatment is rarely afforded to prisoners captured in the conflict. Over the years, vast areas of the country have been declared virtual "free-fire" zones under a draconian counter-insurgency programme, known as the "Four Cuts", which was devised by Burmese army commanders in the 1960s to try and divide insurgent groups from civilian supporters.[4] All such practices, it should be stressed, are in violation of Common Article 3 of the Geneva Conventions (which applies to situations of internal conflict), under which all parties to a conflict are obliged to provide care to both civilian victims and prisoners.[5]

Since 1988, this obsessive secrecy about the impact of some of Asia's least reported conflicts has begun to dissipate. In part, this has been in response to the upsurge in international media interest that followed the events of 1988, when an estimated 10,000 students and other democracy activists fled from Rangoon and other urban areas into territory controlled by armed ethnic minority forces after the SLORC took power. Fierce battles were frequently witnessed by foreign journalists along the Thai and Chinese borders between 1988 and 1992. At the same time, as growing numbers of refugees fled the fighting, serious international concern was also raised over the plight of the civilian victims of the war by organizations such as Amnesty International and Asia Watch (now Human Rights Watch/Asia).[6]

However, changing international awareness of the scale of Burma's humanitarian disaster can also be attributed to an important shift in government policy under the SLORC. This followed the unexpected collapse, due to ethnic mutinies, of the country's largest insurgent force, the Communist Party of Burma, in 1989. The first evidence of this change came in January 1990 when General Saw Maung, the former SLORC Chairman, publicly admitted that the real death toll in over 40 years of armed conflict "would reach as high as millions".[7] Since this landmark statement, the SLORC has offered peace talks — with the added enticement of development aid — to all of Burma's armed opposition ethnic forces for the first time since 1963.

All the cease-fires agreed to date, it should be emphasized, have been purely military, with no serious political issues discussed, while the SLORC proceeds with its National Convention process in Rangoon.[8] Similarly, the cornerstone of the SLORC's new ethnic policy is the Border Areas Development Programme (BADP), which technically co-ordinates projects between the Health Ministry and other government departments, but remains under direct military control. This has led to some very different claims over what is actually being achieved. For example, since the BADP's establishment in 1989, the SLORC claims to have invested over US$ 400 million (2,842 million kyats[9]) on development initiatives in ethnic minority regions, while opposition groups claim that most of this expenditure has been on buildings and roads, with precious little being spent on health projects where there is local participation in decision-making. Moreover, the SLORC continues to try and restrict all contacts between international aid agencies and ethnic minority forces, which actually control many of these lands (see Chapter 5).

Nonetheless, after a slow beginning, the peace process has begun to gather momentum and, since 1990, the first UN and other international visitors in decades have been allowed to travel to several war-torn areas of the country. Currently, 17 of the 20 largest armed opposition groups in Burma, with over 50,000 troops under arms, have cease-fires with the SLORC.[10] Of equal importance, the SLORC finally acceded to the Geneva Conventions on the Protection of the Victims of War in 1992. Previously, Burma was one of just four countries not to have signed.

Thus, with the SLORC's most recent cease-fire with the 15,000-strong Mong Tai Army (MTA) of Khun Sa in January 1996, the situation is extremely delicately poised. As fighting comes to a halt, opposition groups and community leaders are hoping that the establishment of peace will allow serious attention to be paid to the many health and humanitarian problems caused by the war, including the welfare of refugees and the internally displaced, the effects of the indiscriminate use of land-mines, and the conscription of children as soldiers.[11]

Tragically, however, continuing injuries and casualties are still being reported in different regions of the country, even in some areas where cease-fires have been agreed. On 21 March 1995, for example, a cease-fire was signed by the Karenni National Progressive Party (KNPP) in Loikaw, the Kayah State capital, in which the SLORC reportedly agreed to stop using local civilians for forced labour or portering. However, just three months later, seven badly wounded porters were rushed by local medics to hospital in neighbouring Thailand after being ordered to walk ahead of government troops through a KNPP minefield. As local clashes over trade and territory escalated, few observers were surprised when full-scale fighting broke out again in January 1996. Similarly, in May 1996 there were reports of a number of villagers being shot dead and many villages destroyed after the SLORC ordered the forced relocation into government-held areas of over 300 villages in the central and southern Shan State, in an attempt to take advantage of the military vacuum caused by the MTA cease-fire and the apparent defection of the MTA leader, Khun Sa, to Rangoon.

At the same time, there has also been no let-up in reports of gross human rights violations where formal cease-fires have yet to be agreed. In November 1995, for example, the UN Special Rapporteur to Myanmar presented evidence to the UN General Assembly of "torture, arbitrary killings, rapes" and other "atrocious acts", particularly against members of ethnic minorities, women, peasants and "other peaceful civilians who do not have enough money to avoid mistreatment by bribing".[12] The Special Rapporteur provided documentation from the Karen State in the south to the Chin State in Burma's far north but, like similar such allegations in the past, they elicited no substantive response from the SLORC or any official investigations. Nor are details of the Special Rapporteur's reports published in the state media.

Equally serious, during recent fighting, government censorship and political propaganda have been employed to help foment division among ethnic minority forces and further the SLORC's military objectives. Indeed, many ethnic minority leaders believe that governmental misuse of the media could ultimately jeopardize the success of the entire peace process. The health implications are enormous. Across the country, millions of displaced people hope that, at last, they may soon be able to return to develop their homelands. However, other than the occasional announcement of meetings, much of what occurs during the peace discussions, and their security implications for the local people, remain shrouded in official secrecy. Moreover, while all sides have agreed on the need for caution after so many years of bloodshed and ill will, some opposition groups allege that the government's manipulation of the media over the past three years has led to further destitution and loss of life, even while *Tatmadaw* officials are publicly advocating peace.

Such fears were dramatically illustrated in early 1995 by the SLORC's response to a mutiny by several hundred Buddhist soldiers from the Karen National Union (KNU) in south-east Burma. Following months of growing acrimony, the dissident troops finally rebelled against the KNU's predominantly Christian leadership in December 1994 under the guidance of Sayadaw U Thuzana, a local Buddhist abbot.[13] However, even though it had already engaged in the first stages of peace talks with the KNU, the SLORC seized the opportunity to lend immediate support to the rebels, providing them with food and weaponry to help them establish a new armed force, the Democratic Karen Buddhist Organization (DKBO). Then, using the DKBO militia as cover, the SLORC unilaterally broke off the cease-fire offer to the KNU and launched a full-scale offensive, overrunning the KNU's headquarters at Mannerplaw.

As so often in Burma's troubled past, the main victims have once again been civilians. Taking advantage of the divisions within the KNU, new "Four Cuts" operations were launched in 1995 in Karen-inhabited areas of Kyaukkyi, Nyaunglebin, Toungoo, Papun and Tavoy districts, well away from the DKBO rebellion. Government troops reportedly burned down villages, conscripted porters and extrajudicially executed villagers.[14] Eventually, as a result of the KNU split, several thousand Buddhist Karen refugees did return into areas where the DKBO is active, but many more villagers fled the Burmese army advance, bringing the total number of Karen refugees in Thailand to well past the 70,000 mark.

As has long been usual, day-to-day conditions in the war zones remained unreported in the Burmese media throughout all these developments. But in spreading confusion and fear, Karen community leaders contend that the role of the press has been critical. In early 1995, the *New Light of Myanmar* carried a 33-part series of articles entitled, "Whither KNU?", denigrating the Karen nationalist movement with a carefully-woven mixture of fact and fiction. Most KNU soldiers and Karens are, in fact, Buddhists, but the main thrust of these articles was to accuse the KNU's president, Bo Mya, and Christian zealots within the KNU movement of plotting anti-Buddhist discrimination and atrocities. To ensure that these allegations reached the widest possible audience, many of these reports were also carried on state radio (including the newly-inaugurated Myawaddy station of the Burmese Armed Forces or *Tatmadaw*), and in June 1995 they were reproduced in book form in both Burmese and English-language versions.[15]

The attempt to foster the Karen split took a further serious turn when the refugee population in Thailand also appeared to be targeted. Pamphlets and letters were circulated, in the name of the DKBO, in villages and Karen refugee camps along the Thai-Burma border, ordering all Buddhists among the refugees to return to Burma and threatening reprisals against any families who did not immediately move to a resettlement area around U Thuzana's headquarters at Myaing Gyi Ngu. "Those who still remain in the refugee camps will be considered as anti-Buddhist KNU and will be destroyed," warned one widely-circulated letter.[16]

These threats were then followed by a campaign of cross-border raids by DKBO units, which are still continuing, on official refugee camps inside the Thai border, in which at least 30 Karens or Thai nationals (reportedly including three border police) were killed and dozens of refugees were kidnapped back to Burma.[17] In the process, three refugee camps were destroyed and several former KNU officials were taken prisoner, including 71-year-old ex-Brigadier-General Tu Roo, who was executed on the spot by DKBO guerrillas when he proved too ill to walk. Warnings and accusations have also been made by the DKBO against foreign aid workers, which were echoed in the *New Light of Myanmar* when it accused Jack Dunford, a British charity worker who chairs the Burmese Border Consortium co-ordinating international relief, of being a "spy" responsible for en-gineering "an alliance" between the KNU and the MTA of Khun Sa.[18]

And yet, despite frequent eyewitness reports of close collabora-tion between DKBO troops and government forces, the SLORC has continued to deny any involvement other than to "provide security" for local inhabitants and the breakaway Buddhist army.[19] Indeed, as elsewhere in the Shan State, the SLORC appears quite deliberately to use such proxy or local militia forces as the DKBO as a means of denying any responsibility itself for such violations.[20] In a formal reply to the UN Special Rapporteur to Myanmar in July 1995, the SLORC Foreign Ministry claimed that, since the government "should not be held responsible for alleged human rights violations" beyond its control, "the Government of Myanmar is unable to comprehend your concern about the current situation along the Thai/Myanmar border".[21] DKBO officers, however, were not so circumspect in the one interview they gave to Thai journalists at the border. "We have attacked and razed the camps. If we did not do so, then the refugees would not return home," argued a Captain Tu Na. "All will have to return."[22]

All such attacks on non-combatants are in complete contraven-tion of the Geneva Conventions which the SLORC signed amidst much fanfare for the international community in 1992. Common Article 3 of the Geneva Conventions, which applies in situations of internal armed conflict, not only requires health care for the sick and the wounded, but it expressly forbids torture, murder or the taking of hostages, stating that "persons taking no active part in the hostilities, including members of armed forces who have laid down their arms," shall "in all circumstances be treated humanely". Moreover, Common Article 3 clearly obliges all parties to the conflict, including groups such as the DKBO or KNU, to adhere to these minimum standards of internal conflict.[23]

Somewhat unexpectedly, then, at the end of a year of such conflict and suffering, in late 1995 the SLORC re-opened the offer of peace talks with the KNU and, in October, government representatives began a series of meetings with KNU leaders, including Bo Mya. As in the other war zones, there appeared to be leaders on both sides who wanted to bring an end to so many years of fighting, but local refugees and inhabitants still watched the situation with great caution.

If any further reminder was needed of the continuing dangers, during December 1995 and January 1996 the DKBO resumed attacks on the Karen refugee camps. On 2 December, for example, three refugees, Ka Ka Per, Ka Lar and a middle-aged schoolteacher, Saw Wah, were shot and killed at a funeral service in Shoklo refugee camp. Then, in January, the attacks were turned against foreign aid workers. "Where are the foreign doctors?" demanded DKBO guerrillas in a night-time raid on Shoklo.[24] Dr François Nosten and an Australian colleague, who run an internationally-renowned malaria research programme supported by Mahidol University in Bangkok (Thailand) and Oxford University (UK), narrowly escaped by hiding for the night in a bunker, but Dr Nosten's malaria clinic and a nearby MSF hospital were looted of both medicines and equipment. Having failed in this attempt, the DKBO offered a US$ 400 reward for help in the capture of any foreign aid worker.[25]

The response of the Thai government, which appeared more preoccupied with improving relations with the SLORC government (see 6.2 below), was to step up security and plan to close yet another camp, moving all 9,405 inhabitants of Shoklo further away from the border. Thus, far from finding safe sanctuary abroad, for these victims of war more upset has been imposed upon already badly-disrupted lives.

6.2 Refugees and the Internal Displacement of Civilians

Civilian displacement, due to armed conflict and other political reasons, has long been one of the least recognized social and health problems in Burma. Millions of local inhabitants have undergone this bitter experience since Burma's independence in 1948. In general, people who are currently displaced can be divided into three main groups: civilians internally displaced due to war; those forcibly relocated under government resettlement programmes; and refugees (including some deemed as migrants[26]) in neighbouring countries. There are considerable difficulties involved in providing effective health care to all three groups. Burmese society today is in a state of enormous social flux. Nevertheless, each category has been the subject of increasing international concern over the past few years — and not simply over violations of human rights. Worldwide experience has warned that displaced peoples are especially at risk from such serious health problems as malnutrition, malaria, cholera, dysentery and, in some cases, narcotics and even AIDS, all of which have the most damaging impact on the health of the nation. Although marginalized, the health status of these most vulnerable groups cannot be divorced from the health problems of the rest of society.

The most neglected are the internally-displaced people in the war zones. Estimates vary widely over the numbers affected, but community leaders believe that they number well over one million today, especially ethnic minority Karens, Karennis, Mons, Kachins, Shans, Palaungs and Was. Many live in remote forests and mountains in the borderland areas, but there are also large concentrations of displaced peoples around ethnic minority towns as well as numerous villagers who have been forcibly relocated into "strategy villages" during government counter-insurgency operations. In the northern Shan State, for example, community leaders estimate that up to half the local population has either moved into the towns, been internally displaced in the mountains or has fled to the border since fighting first erupted in the 1960s. In the northern Wa region alone, there are currently estimated to be 70,000 inhabitants of 32 camps in areas controlled by the United Wa State Party along the border with China.

Similarly, in the Kachin State to the north, the Kachin Independence Organization (KIO) has calculated that, despite its 1994 cease-fire with the SLORC, in late 1995 there were still over 60,000 displaced people in the hills, a further 10,000 refugees in camps along the China border, as well as over 60,000 villagers in relocation villages under government military control.[27]

For the moment, all such groups remain beyond the reach of effective international health care or aid, due to a combination of both governmental intransigence and military tension. The UK-based NGO, Health Unlimited, has recently begun the first ever child immunization project in KIO-controlled areas of the Kachin State (by approaching from the border) and, like MSF, Aide Médicale Internationale and several other Western NGOs, has in the past been involved in small health projects in the Thai border region. But the great majority of Burma's displaced peoples are still having to be self-reliant, despite the announcement of the SLORC's Border Areas Development Programme. The little investment to date has been on infrastructure and buildings, with few health-training or educational programmes. There also remain vast areas where, due to conflict, government authorities have never had any access.

For their part, armed opposition groups are sometimes able to provide emergency food or shelter, depending on their strengths and capabilities. Over the years, ethnic minority parties such as the KIO and KNU have trained many local health workers, but away from military camps medical provision is minimal and there are only a handful of qualified doctors in territories that they control. As a result, in large areas many serious health problems have long remained untreated. Community health workers report that, in most districts, malaria is usually the major health problem, but illnesses such as tuberculosis, tetanus, typhoid, diarrhoea, pneumonia, hepatitis and cholera are also a constant threat. In addition, in north-east Burma there is now increasing concern about heroin addiction and the recent spread of HIV/AIDS.

These grim health conditions, however, are rarely monitored or reported either in Burma or the world outside. Every year thousands of civilians and villagers die in Burma's borderland areas during health emergencies that attract only occasional public attention. In August 1993, for example, Chinese doctors crossed into UWSP-controlled areas of the eastern Shan State after an outbreak of cholera in two displaced persons' camps. Here they diagnosed and treated over 940 cases. In the same period, however, Karen villagers in south-east Burma and Palaung villagers in the northern Shan State were not so fortunate as to receive treatment. Reports later emerged of several hundred deaths in a number of localized outbreaks of sickness which, despite allegations that the Burmese army was using biological weapons, were generally accepted to be attributable to cholera.[28]

Although less severe, many of the same basic health problems often afflict the second displaced population in Burma: civilians forcibly relocated under government resettlement programmes. Resettlement policies have existed in Burma since the 1950s, and in 1985 the former BSPP government began to develop several new relocation areas around Rangoon. However, the scale of these relocations has accelerated rapidly under the SLORC which, opposition groups allege, has used such programmes as a form of social control after many workers in downtown urban areas took part in the 1988 democracy protests. According to an unpublished report by Habitat (the UN Centre for Human Settlements), by 1990 1.5 million people or 4 per cent of Burma's population at that time had been affected by displacement, including 16 per cent of the urban population. Of this number, over 250,000 people have been compulsorily moved from Rangoon to the satellite new towns of Hlaingthayar and Shwepyithar since 1989.

Conditions vary widely at many of these new settlements, and while there has been some demand (and land speculation) for housing at better-located sites, in other areas living conditions are extremely poor, especially in the early stages of resettlement. Not only are such illnesses as dengue haemorrhagic fever and diarrhoea common due to inadequate drainage and sanitary facilities, but little or no consideration has been given to the social and health implications of the break-up of so many long-standing communities. These communities were already poor, but forced relocation and poor housing conditions away from the main job centres have contributed to their high levels of unemployment, poverty, malnutrition, family separation, and increases in illegal abortions and sexually-transmitted diseases.

Since many of these factors can be attributed to resettlement policy, the extremely poor health conditions in many relocation areas provide another major dilemma to international aid agencies considering setting up programmes inside Burma. To date, it has been in some of these very resettlement sites that government authorities have been willing to allow foreign organizations to work, ostensibly in the cause of promoting social progress and development. Considerable delays continue on granting permission and issuing Memoranda of Understanding before official aid work can begin. But in 1992, while other agencies were still hesitating, the first two international NGOs to enter Burma after 1988, MSF (Netherlands) and World Vision, considered the health conditions so serious as to warrant their immediate institution of an array of health studies and programmes in the Rangoon satellite towns of Hlaingthayar and Shwepyithar (MSF) and Dawpon, Hlaingthayar and South Dagon, as well as one new town in Mandalay (World Vision). Particular concentration has been given to nutrition, health education, AIDS-awareness and the health of women and children in the first independent NGO health projects begun in Burma in decades. However, one of the primary causes of such poor health in these areas — the government's resettlement policy itself — remains unaddressed.

Similar dilemmas surround the treatment of the third displaced persons group: the country's huge population of refugees and exiles living abroad. Burma has produced one of the largest refugee populations in Asia. According to official government figures, in January 1996 there were 93,252 refugees (mostly Karens, Karennis and Mons) in Thailand, some 50,000 Muslim refugees in Bangladesh (following the repatriation of over 190,000 refugees in 1994-1995), as well as an estimated 60,000 refugees in India and China.

These figures, however, do not reflect the long-term exodus of many other victims of Burma's political turmoil. This has important health implications for all of Burma's neighbours. In the present era of HIV/AIDS and increasing drug resistance to malaria, health workers need access to the community and unrestricted ability to conduct research if the spread of a whole variety of viral or communicable diseases is to be addressed. In Thailand, for example, a recent governmental study put the total number of refugees and illegal migrants from Burma at over 350,000, causing Thai officials to express concern for their country's "national security" as well as social, political and economic development.[29] However, although subsistence food and medical aid is provided for refugees in the official camps[30], the urgent health problems of the majority of this largely transient population, many of whom secretly travel backwards and forwards to Burma, are not being addressed in any systematic way. In August 1995, for example, the Thai Deputy-Minister of Public Health warned that an estimated 60 per cent of all malaria cases being treated in Thailand were among "illegal immigrants", most of whom came from Burma or Cambodia.[31] Equally serious, the AIDS pandemic in south-east Asia now poses an even greater threat, with health officials recently reporting that over 200 AIDS sufferers from Burma were being treated in public hospitals in Thailand's Mae Hong Son province alone (see Chapter 7).[32]

For the moment, however, the main focus of international concern is the humanitarian treatment and future repatriation of all refugees, an issue which is likely to gain momentum with the recent Karenni, Mon and Mong Tai Army cease-fires. For many years, the Thai government has had a largely tolerant attitude to refugees from Burma, but there are growing indications that official thinking is beginning to change. In part, this is due to the sheer numbers involved, but it is also part of a long-term plan by the Thai government to normalize relations with the SLORC in order that Burma may become a member of the Association of South East Asian Nations (ASEAN). In 1995, as a first step, the SLORC signed ASEAN's "Treaty of Amity and Cooperation" and, despite the DKBO attacks across the border, Thailand's new policy of "constructive engagement" has survived.

As a result, exiles from Burma are coming under increasing pressure from different Thai authorities. Already many Mon, Karenni and Karen refugees have been removed into remote border areas (sometimes in response to DKBO attacks[33]), despite the many health and other hardships this has entailed. Meanwhile, in the past three years, thousands of Burmese migrants have been arrested who have been found living illegally or working outside the camps.[34] In one notorious example, a severely-handicapped Mon refugee, Maung Kyan, who had lost his eyesight and both his arms in a land-mine explosion, was arrested in April 1995 after travelling to Bangkok for essential medical treatment. He was then held with his family in the Immigration Detention Centre for over two months before being released, after an international campaign for his liberty, into the "Safe-Area" camp near

Ratchaburi, which was set up in 1992 by the Ministry of the Interior for exiled Burmese students.[35]

The prospect of such publicity, however, or modern health care, is not available to the many refugees and exiles now facing repatriation to Burma. Both the Thai and SLORC governments have resisted any international monitoring presence. Indeed, although it has granted "persons of concern" status to over 2,000 Burmese students in Bangkok, the UNHCR has, to date, never become involved in the plight of refugees at the Burma border, although in April 1995 it did request the Thai National Security Council to allow some form of monitoring presence to be set up following the DKBO's attacks on refugee camps.[36] This request was refused, although reportedly repeated by the UNHCR in January 1996.

With the return and reintegration of Mon refugees now under way, the Mon National Relief Committee (MNRC) has also expressed concern about the future provision of health and development aid, as well as about protection from forced labour and other human rights abuses.[37] During early 1996, the MNRC oversaw — without any official international monitoring — the repatriation of an estimated 18,000 Mon refugees into territory controlled by the New Mon State Party, which had agreed a cease-fire with the SLORC in June 1995. MNRC officials, however, remain concerned that the cease-fire agreement specifically precluded — at the SLORC's insistence — returning refugees and internally-displaced civilians from receiving cross-border assistance to help resettlement once the refugees had returned into Burma. Previously, rice and other humanitarian relief had been provided to the refugees by the Burmese Border Consortium of international NGOs. But any further aid, both Thai and SLORC officials have insisted, must come from the Burmese government side.

In November 1995, in an initial response to such concerns, a UNHCR delegation visited Rangoon to discuss establishing a monitoring presence inside the Burmese border to ensure a "safe and dignified" return of refugees from Thailand.[38] Following the failure of this mission, another delegation visited in March 1996, but still no agreement was reached. As a result, many refugees remain unconvinced over the security of repatriation procedures. Indeed, the experiences of refugee populations around Burma's borders has not given much grounds for optimism. In September 1994, for example, thousands of

Chin refugees and exiles living in Mizoram in north-east India were suddenly rounded up by police and handed over to the SLORC authorities who, according to local reports, promptly arrested many of them. In China, too, over 30,000 refugees are still estimated to be living in borderland communities, and in 1995 the KIO eventually tried to begin a resettlement programme for 10,000 Kachin refugees, using its own limited funds and resources in one of the world's most inaccessible borderland regions.[39]

As a repatriation model, however, most international attention has remained focused on the repatriation to Burma of Muslim refugees who had fled to Bangladesh. In 1991-1992, Burma's Rakhine State was the scene of a major refugee exodus for the second time in 14 years, when over 260,000 members of the Muslim minority (sometimes known as Rohingyas) fled into Bangladesh amidst widespread reports of human rights violations by the local Burmese military and *Na Sa Ka* border police. According to eyewitness testimony, forced labour, forced relocations, torture and extrajudicial executions were widespread.[40] Just as in 1978, disinformation in the government press played a crucial role in exacerbating religious fears while hiding the real reasons. Instead, the SLORC variously blamed the exodus on "scaremongering" by small groups of *Mujahid* extremists or illegal Bengali immigrants. "The Rohingya problem is no more than the problem of unregistered illegal immigrants," claimed the *Working People's Daily* in January 1992.

Under a bilateral agreement between the SLORC and Bangladesh governments, an estimated 50,000 refugees were sent back to Burma in late 1992 without an international monitoring presence and amidst widespread allegations that the refugees were being forced to return against their will. Following international pressure, however, the SLORC appeared to relent and a monitored repatriation programme was eventually arranged in a Memorandum of Understanding between the UNHCR and SLORC government in November 1993. In 1994 the first repatriations began under UNHCR auspices and, according to the UNHCR, its initial US$ 34 million programme has since changed emphasis from "repatriation" to "resettlement" and "reintegration".[41] By January 1996, over 194,000 refugees had officially returned, leaving a further 50,000 refugees in Bangladesh, who were generally considered to be refugees identified with opposition groups or individuals, separated from their families, whom the local SLORC authorities wanted to check more closely.

Disagreements, however, have continued at every stage of the repatriation process, especially over the level of protection afforded to members of a minority group who have twice been driven from their homes within 14 years. In this respect, the level of information supplied to the refugees and the access of neutral observers to the resettlement procedures are critical in assessing whether the repatriations have been conducted under universal standards of human rights protection.

Initial concerns centred on how voluntary the repatriations actually were. Not for the first time, the analysis by UN agencies in Burma differed markedly from that of international NGOs. The US Committee for Refugees, Refugees International and MSF, for example, all published reports indicating that not only were refugees pressurized by the Bangladeshi authorities — including by food deprivation and beatings — to leave their 20 makeshift camps, but they were not adequately informed of their rights to reject repatriation under international humanitarian law.[42] Indeed, MSF was so concerned by the impending repatriations that it conducted its own "awareness survey", which showed that 65 per cent of the families questioned did not know of their right to refuse repatriation.[43] Of special concern to MSF was a change in UNHCR policy in July 1994, from one of individual interviews and "information sessions" for refugees to mass "voluntary" registrations for repatriation; this brought about a dramatic rise in the numbers officially willing to return — from 23 per cent in one camp survey to around 95 per cent overall.[44] Not surprisingly, if such methods were allowed to pass unchallenged, MSF feared that they could set a precedent for similar mass repatriations as "solutions" to other refugee emergencies around the world.

Further concerns have followed the treatment of refugees upon their return, and particularly whether the refugees' much-documented fears of persecution have been properly addressed in the absence of substantive political reform in Burma.[45] Article 33 of the 1951 Convention Relating to the Status of Refugees expressly forbids the returning of refugees to territories where their lives or freedom could be "threatened" on account of "race, religion, nationality, membership of a particular social group or political opinion". For its part, the

UNHCR, with the presence of 15 international officers inside Burma, has said that it is satisfied with the SLORC's guarantees of safety.[46]

Opposition groups, however, have not been reassured. Not only have the returnees been resettled in remote border areas — and, sometimes, away from their original homes — but they have been issued by the Burmese authorities with temporary identity cards that do not grant full citizenship rights. Moreover, foreign journalists and health workers have been barred from visiting the resettlement region independently. Indeed, recent travellers report that security surveillance is intensive, returnees are not allowed to make long journeys without official permission, and in many areas UN and international NGO workers are not allowed to travel without a military escort. During March and April 1996, a further 3,000 Muslim refugees (700 of whom were pushed back by the Bangladeshi authorities) fled into Bangladesh, even while the repatriation and resettlement process was continuing. Equally concerning, the practice of forced labour, which was a major reason for the exodus in the first place, continues to be widespread. This is acknowledged by the UNHCR, which has made the dubious claim to have reduced "the burden for both the local population and returnees" to a maximum of four days of work a month per family after intervening with the authorities.[47]

That the UNHCR has negotiated with the government over the frequency of an inhumane labour practice, which has been repeatedly condemned by the UN General Assembly, the International Labour Organization and other world bodies, does much to exemplify the difficulties international aid agencies face in trying to ensure the most basic health and humanitarian protection for the Burmese peoples. The SLORC itself has always been inconsistent in its response to forced labour concerns, which have long had a detrimental impact on the health of the people. In 1995, for example, though publicly denying that forced labour existed, SLORC officials privately told the UN Special Rapporteur to Myanmar that a "Secret Directive" had been issued to "discourage" its further use.[48] Yet no real evidence has been found to support this claim. The Special Rapporteur was later presented with two recent directives, marked "secret" and promulgated by the office of the SLORC Chairman, which warned regional military authorities that the local populace must be paid for work on both "national development" and "irrigation" projects; the practice of unpaid labour must "stop".[49] However, as the Special Rapporteur pointed out, neither of the directives abrogated existing legislation under the 1908 Village Act and Towns Act, which authorized the use of forced labour under certain conditions. Equally serious, the Special Rapporteur noted that:

> Several months after their publication, these directives are still not public and therefore not accessible to those to whom they would apply and to those protecting the rights of the persons accused of breaking the laws.[50]

Nonetheless, as a test case, the work of the UNHCR in trying to "anchor" Muslim returnees back in the Rakhine State has provided a rare glimpse of health conditions in at least one ethnic minority region of the country. In rural areas of Maungdaw and Buthidaung, for example, the UNHCR has uncovered a ratio of only one doctor to nearly 100,000 local inhabitants, as compared to one doctor to 1,600 refugees in the camps in Bangladesh and one doctor to 12,500 people within Burma nationally.[51] Equally stark, 90 per cent of local residents are illiterate and only 15 per cent of children in the returnee areas attend government schools, which are under-funded and generally poorly-run.

In response, the UNHCR has begun a wide-ranging "reintegration" programme that focuses on health, water, sanitation, education, transportation and community service projects. In keeping with the UNDP's guidelines that programmes in Burma should be run at the grass roots level, some of these projects are being run in conjunction with the MRC and MMCWA (community services) and others (water and sanitation) with the UN World Food Programme and the French NGO, Action Internationale Contre la Faim. In the process, over 400 village wells or ponds are being built and 41 schools renovated. The UNHCR also plans to spend a further US$ 23.9 million in the resettlement process during 1996-1997.

These emergency programmes undoubtedly help sustain displaced peoples in a time of great need. However, the agencies' necessarily close involvement with the government's chosen authorities is very problematic. The question still remains of how a shift can be made from emergency provision to long-term development based on genuine local participation. Returnees, for example, privately complain about the lack of trained medical staff who speak their language, understand their customs and are sensitive to the culture of Muslim women. Indeed, the SLORC authorities hand-pick all local officials and headmen.

Present programmes of international assistance are thus based on expediency and humanitarian need, with an emphasis on what the UNDP describes as Quick Impact Projects (QUIPS). However, for sustainable development and health initiatives to really take root, the need remains as acute as ever for social, political and educational reforms, in which the democratic right to participation is restored to the local people.

6.3 The Health of Prisoners and Detainees

The treatment of prisoners and detainees in Burma is another major area of health and human rights concern. In the war zones, reports of the summary arrest, torture or extrajudicial executions of both villagers and suspected insurgents have long been commonplace (see 6.1 above). However, over the years there have also been continuing allegations of human rights violations against detainees in prison, which have a particular impact on their health. Amnesty International, for example, has identified 20 detention centres across the country where "brutal interrogation" has taken place.[52] Documented methods of torture include various forms of water torture, electric shock treatment and beatings. Another persistent complaint has been the lack of adequate medical provision for political prisoners and that families face obstructions in sending medicines or other essential supplies into prisons.[53] In a further act of deprivation, although the prison authorities say that reading and writing materials are allowed, there are former political prisoners who claim that, in practice, they are frequently denied.

After the SLORC assumed power in 1988, several thousand students and democracy activists were detained in a succession of security clampdowns by the authorities. Former detainees interviewed by ARTICLE 19, many of whom were still suffering from ill-health, reported the widespread and systematic use of food and sleep deprivation, beatings and the denial of adequate medical care. In the course of such ill-treatment, health problems such as bronchitis, pneumonia or heart conditions have often become chronic, and at least 16 political prisoners are known to have died between 1988 and 1995. Since there is no mechanism for independent investigation, the exact circumstances of most of these deaths are still unclear, but they have included Maung Thawka (U Ba Thaw), Chairman of Burma's Writers Association, U Maung Ko, the NLD workers' leader, U Oo Tha Tun, a parliamentary candidate and Rakhine historian, and three leaders of the left-wing People's Progressive Party, U Khin Sein, U Nyo Win and U Khin Maung Myint.[54]

In a change of public presentation since April 1992, when General Than Shwe replaced General Saw Maung as SLORC Chairman, the existence of "political prisoners" in Burma has occasionally been admitted by the authorities, and over 2,000 detainees have been released under SLORC Declaration 11/92. In addition, in 1993-1994 the UN Special Rapporteur to Myanmar was permitted brief access to a number of political prisoners in Insein jail on his official visits to the country, including the student leader, Min Ko Naing, and the NLD figures, former-General Tin Oo and Dr Aung Khin Sint, both of whom have since been released.

During 1995, however, the Special Rapporteur was once again denied permission to meet with prisoners, and other prisons and prisoners have remained strictly off-limits to outside visitors, despite repeated requests for access by both the UN Special Rapporteur and the ICRC.[55] Allegations of health and human rights abuses, nevertheless, continue to be reported, in private, by former prisoners. In February 1996, for example, the Special Rapporteur presented testimony to the UN Commission on Human Rights of gross overcrowding in prisons, including a two floor dormitory in Insein jail, measuring 60 feet by 40, in which up to 250 women were held, including 30 children and newborn babies with their mothers. Due to inadequate food, the mortality rate amongst newborn children was reportedly "very high".[56]

Another concern is the health treatment of prisoners who are compelled to work as porters in the war zones or on government construction sites. Across the country, chain-gangs of labourers are an everyday sight. But in the past few years large numbers of prison labourers are reported to have died in working conditions of great hardship, especially in the ethnic minority borderlands where medical treatment is minimal and malaria, dysentery and other potentially fatal diseases are endemic. "There are many prisoners that are dying," a Christian pastor told Amnesty International in 1992 after witnessing prison chain-gangs working on the Myitkyina-Sumprabum-Putao highway in the Kachin State.[57] Many more prisoners were also killed during heavy fighting with the KNU around Mannerplaw in early 1992, having been conscripted as front-line porters from jails all over the country. More recently, the ABSDF has claimed that over 100 prison inmates died in one year from hunger and lack of proper medical care at the Boke Pyin labour camp in southern Burma.[58]

The acute problem of securing access to prisoners by independent visitors, which can provide a crucial means of health protection, was further demonstrated in June 1995 when the ICRC decided to pull out of Burma. The ICRC, which is charged under the Geneva Conventions with visiting prisoners of war and other detainees, took this extraordinary decision in protest at the SLORC's continued refusal to accept three key "customary procedures" that the ICRC insists upon: the right to interview prisoners without witnesses, to see all prisoners and prisons in any part of the country, and to have a guaranteed right to revisit any prisoner. "To have some credibility we cannot go just once, we need to follow up visits every few months," one official explained. "We also have to see those prisoners in private, without security officials present."[59] As a result, the ICRC office (opened in 1986) was closed down, an artificial limb programme for war victims handed over to the Health Ministry and Myanmar Red Cross, and training classes about the Geneva Conventions for military officers, which had been started after the SLORC's signing of the Conventions in 1992, were stopped altogether.

With the ICRC's withdrawal, there is thus even more concern in Burma over the treatment of prisoners and detainees. This was further heightened by a new crack-down that began on political prisoners in Insein jail in November 1995. In response, the wives of 36 such prisoners reportedly wrote to the Ministry for Home Affairs complaining of a deterioration in the health of their husbands after a new punishment regime, including the denial of medical attention and meetings with relatives, had been introduced. NLD supporters and student democracy activists appeared to be singled out, including U Win Tin,

Vice-Chairman of Burma's Writers Association, U Myo Myint Nyein, a magazine editor, Monywa Tin Shwe, a lawyer, and U Saw Naing Naing and Dr Zaw Myint, NLD MPs-elect for Pazundaung and Henzada-2 respectively. According to NLD sources, food and drink were being restricted and the prisoners moved to military dog cells, where they had to sleep on the floor without blankets.

Details of the individual charges brought against each prisoner remain unclear, but the prisoners concerned were alleged to have been found in possession of anti-government literature and materials. These included three hidden radio sets, a secret newsletter that had been circulating in the prison, and a copy of a letter addressed to the UN Special Rapporteur to Myanmar, signed by several prisoners, which described prison conditions. Eventually on 28 March 1996, 21 of the prisoners received additional jail terms of anywhere between five and 12 years under the Penal Code and Section 5(j) of the Emergency Provisions Act for behaviour which might disrupt the "stability of the Union". Their alleged "crime", it appeared, was to have tried to communicate news of the harsh conditions of their imprisonment to the UN Special Rapporteur to Myanmar. In an international appeal, Amnesty International expressed concern that they may have been sentenced "solely for exercising their rights to 'Contact with the outside world' as provided for in Articles 37 and 39 in the UN Standard Minimum Rules for the Treatment of Prisoners".[60]

There are now widespread anxieties over the health and treatment of all political prisoners in Burma's jails. In particular, 65-year-old Win Tin, one of the NLD's founding theoreticians, is known to suffer from chronic spondylitis and, having been originally jailed in 1989 on tendentious charges of involvement in an abortion case, colleagues fear his imprisonment is now being extended indefinitely (see Chapter 5). Similar fears have been expressed over the condition of another detained writer, 29-year-old Dr Ma Thida, who had been working at the Muslim Free Hospital in Rangoon. Serving a 20-year jail sentence under a variety of censorship laws, she has been suffering from tuberculosis and a number of other health ailments (see Chapter 5). Another political prisoner, whose health is giving cause for concern, is Nay Min, a 47-year-old lawyer, who received a 14-year sentence with hard labour in October 1989 under sections (c) and (j) of the 1950 Emergency Provisions Act for allegedly sending "false news" to the BBC. At the time of his arrest, Nay Min was reportedly tortured, but he has since been moved from Insein to Tharawaddy jail, where it is even more difficult to monitor his health and progress.

In ARTICLE 19's view, therefore, it is imperative that the ICRC should be permitted to return to Burma as soon as possible, under the terms of its internationally-recognized mandate, and resume prison inspections, with free and regular private access to all prisoners. In addition, the UN Special Rapporteur to Myanmar should be permitted to continue all aspects of his investigations into the human rights situation in the country, including his visits to prisons.

NOTES

[1] For a discussion, see, M Smith, *Burma: Insurgency and the Politics of Ethnicity* (London and New Jersey: Zed Books, 1991), 100-1.

[2] M Smith, *Ethnic Groups in Burma: Development, Democracy and Human Rights* (London: Anti-Slavery International, 1994), 40, 62.

[3] In 1986, the ICRC opened an office in Rangoon, but did not become involved in independently monitoring the fighting or the question of prisoners of war. Its main work was in the field of artificial limbs. There are absolutely no studies or reliable figures on the plight of prisoners of war in Burma. The KIO, for example, after its 1994 cease-fire with the SLORC, compiled a list of over 6,000 supporters whom it believed had been arrested (and, in some cases, probably killed) by government forces over the past three decades. The list, however, was not handed over to the SLORC since it was believed that it could endanger the security of the KIO movement before a stable peace is established; see ARTICLE 19, *Censorship Prevails* (see Chapter 1, note 4), 9, 34-35.

[4] See e.g., Smith, note 1 above, at 258-262.

[5] See e.g., J-P Lavoyer, "Refugees and Internally Displaced Persons: International Humanitarian Law and the Role of the ICRC", in *International Review of the Red Cross*, March-April 1995, 164-165.

[6] See e.g., Amnesty International, *Myanmar: "No law at all": Human rights violations under military rule* (London: 1992), 17-29.

[7] *Working People's Daily*, 10 Jan. 1990.

[8] ARTICLE 19, *Censorship Prevails*, (see Chapter 1, note 4), 24-29. Del-

egates from some of the earlier cease-fire armies have intermittently attended sessions of the Convention, but the later organizations to sign cease-fires have either been represented as observers only or have taken no part at all.

[9] *Statement by Ambassador U Pe Thein, Representative of the Union of Myanmar on Agenda Item 112 (c), Human Rights Situations and Reports of Special Rapporteurs* (UN General Assembly Third Committee, 30 Nov. 1995), 5; NB, at the real market rate, 2,842 million kyats is worth only US$ 28 million.

[10] United Wa State Party, Myanmar National Democratic Alliance Army (Kokang), National Democracy Alliance Army (eastern Shan State), New Democratic Army (north-east Kachin State), Shan State Army, Palaung State Liberation Party, Kachin Defence Army (northern Shan State), Pao National Organization, Kachin Independence Organization, Shan State Nationalities Liberation Organization, Karenni Nationalities People's Liberation Front, Kayan New Land Party, Kayan Home Guard, Democratic Karen Buddhist Organization, Karenni National Progressive Party, New Mon State Party and Mong Tai Army. Those yet to agree cease-fires in early May 1996 were the Karen National Union, National Socialist Council of Nagaland and Rohingya Solidarity Alliance. Smaller insurgent forces which are still active include the Chin National Front, National Unity Party of Arakan and the ABSDF.

[11] Smith, note 2 above, at 116-121. The use of under age soldiers has been especially common among ethnic minority forces, notably the UWSP, KNU, KNPP and MTA of Khun Sa. See also, Images Asia, *"No Childhood at all":* *A Report about Child Soldiers in Burma* (Chiang Mai, Nov.-Dec. 1995).

[12] *Statement of Mr Yozo Yokota, Special Rapporteur of the Commission on Human Rights on the Situation of Human Rights in Myanmar to the Fiftieth Session of the General Assembly* (27 Nov. 1995), 9. For a more detailed report, see UN General Assembly, *Situation of Human Rights in Myanmar* (see Chapter 2, note 21).

[13] The grievances of the Buddhist mutineers were serious, including anti-Buddhist discrimination as well as gross human rights abuses by a group of KNU officers in the Paan area, who were reportedly responsible for extra-judicial executions and the forced labour of civilians.

[14] See e.g., *The Nation* (Bangkok), 19 Oct. 1995; Amnesty International, *Myanmar Kayin (Karen) State: the Killings Continue* (London: 1996), 1-14.

[15] From January 1996, a new Karen-language radio station called "Thapyay", apparently run by the DKBO with SLORC approval, was also intermittently heard in the Thai border region.

[16] Amnesty International, *Myanmar: "No Place to Hide": Killings, abductions and other abuses against ethnic Karen villagers and refugees* (London: 1995), 10.

[17] Ibid., at 10-21; Human Rights Watch/Asia, *Burma: Abuses Linked to the Fall of Mannerplaw* (New York: 1995), 16-18.

[18] A Resident of Kayin State, *Whither KNU?* (Rangoon: Myawaddy Press, 1995), 57.

[19] See, UN General Assembly, note 12 above, at 17-20, 29. Some attempts at hiding the Burmese army presence have been very unsubtle. For example, after the fall of Mannerplaw a large boundary sign, "SLORC Tactical Command 661", was clearly visible from the Thai border. A few days later, the sign was replaced with "DKBO" in large letters; for picture, see *Burma Issues* (Bangkok), July 1995, 7.

[20] Since the insurgencies began in 1948, the *Tatmadaw* has regularly made use of cease-fires with local rebel commanders as a means of dissipating stronger opposition forces. A number of different militia systems have been developed over the years, including the *Ka Kwe Ye* home guard troops which grew very powerful in the early 1970s, being allowed to take control of much of the opium trade, before they were once again ordered to disband.

[21] UN General Assembly, note 12 above, at 20.

[22] *The Nation* (Bangkok), 1 May 1995.

[23] Human Rights Watch/Asia, note 17 above, at 4-6.

[24] R Moreau, "Doctors Under Fire", *Newsweek*, 19 Feb. 1996.

[25] Throughout early 1996, attacks and robberies by DKBO guerrillas continued across the Thai border. Then, in April, a Dutch couple, who were working as malaria researchers in the refugee camps, were robbed — and the woman raped — by five armed men whom the local Thai authorities claimed were Burmese army soldiers from a 22nd Light Infantry Division unit stationed at Yebu, on the opposite side of the border from the attack. The case is still being investigated; see *Bangkok Post*, 11 April 1996; *The Nation* (Bangkok), 14 April 1996.

[26] In Burma's case, the distinction between refugees, who are recognized under international definitions, and/or migrants is often very difficult to make. During the past three decades, large numbers of Burma's peoples have crossed into neighbouring countries due to fear of persecution as well as the poverty and suffering caused by ethnic and political conflict. Many have avoided local authorities or refugee camps and since found work (mostly illegal, but

sometimes legal) in an exodus which has accelerated since 1988. But while international agencies, such as the UNHCR, strictly reject refugee status where there is a perceived economic motive, many such exiles see themselves as victims of Burma's political troubles and fear enforced return.

[27] See e.g., KIO, *Collective Endeavour: A Report on Reconstruction Activities in Kachin State* (Oct. 1995), 2.

[28] See Chapter 4, note 19.

[29] See e.g., *Bangkok Post*, 22 Jan. 1995.

[30] Since 1984, under an agreement with the Thai Ministry of the Interior, international NGOs have been providing relief aid to the refugees, presently under the aegis of the Burmese Border Consortium (BBC). Malaria and respiratory diseases are the major health problems, but supplementary feeding programmes have also been run by MSF (France) and the Consortium to support vulnerable groups, including underweight children, pregnant women and tuberculosis patients, as well as deal with such persistent health problems as beriberi.

[31] *The Nation* (Bangkok), 16 Aug. 1995.

[32] *Bangkok Post*, 26 Feb. 1995.

[33] In July 1994, a Mon refugee camp at Halockhani just on the Burma side of the Thai border had also been attacked by the Burmese army. In March 1996, attacks were also reported around Karenni refugee camps in Thailand's Mae Hong Son province following fighting with the KNPP across the border.

[34] See e.g., Human Rights Watch/Asia, *The Mon: Persecuted in Burma, Forced out of Thailand* (New York: 1994) and *Abuses against Burmese Refugees in Thailand* (New York: 1992); Amnesty International, *Thailand: Concerns about Treatment of Burmese Refugees* (London: 1991). In early 1996, deportations by the Thai authorities were estimated to be running at around 1,500 per month into a "no-man's land" refugee area straddling the border near Three Pagodas Pass.

[35] *The Nation* (Bangkok), 19 June 1995.

[36] AFP, 26 April 1995.

[37] MNRC, *Regarding the Repatriation Program of Mon Refugees*, 31 Aug. 1995.

[38] *The Nation* (Bangkok), 17 Nov. 1995.

[39] See e.g., KIO, note 27 above.

[40] See e.g., Human Rights Watch/Asia, *Burma: Rape, Forced Labor and Religious Persecution in Northern Arakan* (New York: 1992).

[41] UNHCR, *Return to Myanmar: Repatriating Refugees from Bangladesh*, Information Bulletin, June 1995.

[42] US Committee for Refugees, *The Return of the Rohingya Refugees to Burma: Voluntary Repatriation or Refoulement* (Washington: 1995); Refugees International, *Rohingya Refugees in Bangladesh* (Washington: 1994); MSF, *MSF's concerns on the repatriation of Rohingya refugees from Bangladesh to Burma* (Amsterdam and Paris: 1995).

[43] Ibid., at 4.

[44] Ibid., at 3; UNHCR, note 41 above, at 3.

[45] See e.g., Australian Council for Overseas Aid and Burma NGO Forum, *Repatriation of Burmese Refugees from Thailand and Bangladesh* (Deakin Act, 1996), 6-11.

[46] In June 1995, the UNHCR did nevertheless report that 45 refugees who had returned were being held in detention; see UNHCR, note 41 above, at 4.

[47] Ibid., at 6.

[48] *Statement of Mr Yozo Yokota*, note 12 above, at 8.

[49] UN Economic and Social Council, *Report on the Situation of Human Rights in Myanmar, prepared by Mr Yozo Yokota, Special Rapporteur of the Commission on Human Rights, in accordance with Commission Resolution 1995/72* (Geneva: 5 Feb. 1996), 41-2.

[50] Ibid., at 29. For the most recent update on the Muslim repatriation, see also, Human Rights Watch/Asia, *Burma's Rohingya Muslims: Ending the Cycle of Exodus?* (NewYork: July 1996).

[51] UNHCR, note 41 above, at 7.

[52] Amnesty International, note 6 above, at 13.

[53] Prisoners are allowed visitors for one 15-minute session every two weeks. Medicines, however, have to be handed over to the warders, who then pass them on to the prisoners on what some former detainees claim is often an inconsistent, daily basis.

[54] For descriptions of conditions in prisons, see, Amnesty International, note 6 above, at 14-16, 24; Win Naing Oo, *Cries from Insein: Experiences of a Political Prisoner* (ABSDF, Bangkok: June 1996).

[55] On a visit to Burma in October 1995, the Special Rapporteur went to Insein

and Myitkyina jails but, although he was told that prisoners were in good health, he was not allowed to see any prisoners or inspect their cells.

[56] UN Economic and Social Council, note 49 above, at 23.

[57] Amnesty International, note 6 above, at 20.

[58] ABSDF press release, 22 Jan. 1996.

[59] Reuters, 19 June 1995.

[60] Amnesty International, *Urgent Action*, 2 April 1996. U Win Tin received an additional five years, Myo Myint Nyein seven years, Dr Zaw Myint 12 years, and U Hla Than (another NLD MP-elect) and Tint San (ex-chairperson of Rangoon University Students Union) seven years each.

Chapter 7

AIDS AND NARCOTICS

In recent years, the increasing problems of AIDS and narcotics abuse in Burma have attracted considerable international concern, but no health issues have suffered more from the dearth of accurate field research and data. Epidemic crises in both fields have been allowed to develop against a fatal backdrop of censorship, ignorance, insurgency, governmental inaction and international speculation over the true scale of the problems. Decades of health neglect, however, have inflicted a heavy toll. Not only is Burma the world's largest producer of illicit opium and heroin but, with just 9,885 identified cases of HIV-infection (and 550 of AIDS) in 1995, as compared with WHO estimates of up to 500,000 HIV-carriers, there is no other country in the world with such a vast gap between projections and corroborated figures.[1]

In combating HIV/AIDS, it is, of course, only too easy to be wise after the event. But, as ARTICLE 19 pointed out as long ago as 1991, Burma has long had a number of high-risk factors which make the country a predictable centre for the rapid spread of the disease.[2] In particular, Burma stands out as a country where economic, political and migrational factors have dangerously exacerbated underlying social and health problems. In the global struggle against AIDS, no country can stand isolated.

There is always a danger of prejudice or victimization with generalizations about particular social groups, but international specialists are today agreed that the initial high risk factor behind the spread of HIV in Burma was widespread drug abuse throughout the country's borderland regions. Located on the crossroads between south and southeast Asia, it was mostly intravenous drug users (IDUs) sharing needles to inject heroin from Burma's Golden Triangle region who accounted for the extraordinary explosion in the transmission of HIV/AIDS in the late 1980s. Detailed evidence is lacking from Burma itself, but this pattern of transmission has since been confirmed by studies in neighbouring countries. Burma today is classified by the WHO as one of Asia's "HIV Top Three" along with India and

Thailand, and there are high levels of HIV-infection in all borderland areas where intravenous drug use is prevalent. In China, for example, 70 per cent of all identified HIV-carriers come from Ruili on Burma's border; in India, the small frontier state of Manipur contains 16 per cent of all recorded HIV-carriers; and in Thailand, the incidence of AIDS sky-rocketed throughout the country in the early 1990s, spreading from the border provinces of Chiang Rai, Chiang Mai and Mae Hong Son.[3] In Mae Hong Son province alone, in 1995 public health officials recorded a rate of 18.5 per cent HIV-infection in a random survey of ten villages near the Burma border.[4]

A second initial factor behind the rapid spread in HIV/AIDS is the illicit sex trade between Burma and Thailand. For the past few years, tens of thousands of impoverished girls and young women from Burma have travelled backwards and forwards to Thailand, where many have become prostitutes in the myriad bars, brothels and massage parlours that exist in all of Thailand's main towns. The scale of this secretive trade is massive, with as many as 40,000 Burmese women, many of whom are from ethnic minorities, estimated to be working in Thailand at any one time.[5] The health risks are legion. Recent medical studies have suggested that the probability of HIV-infection is up to ten times greater when the AIDS virus is passed on in conjunction with other sexually transmitted diseases (STDs).[6] Yet such information is not available to the young women from Burma, who do not speak Thai and often work in the poorest brothels, frequently without condom protection. In Burma, too, sex education, condom use and the treatment of STDs are even more scarce, leaving many women extremely vulnerable to infection (see Chapter 8).

The fatal implications for Thailand and its neighbours have not been lost on Thai health workers. Indeed, when 17 out of 19 ethnic Shan teenage prostitutes (none of whom had any knowledge of AIDS) tested HIV-positive after a brothel-raid in Chiang Rai, Mechai Viravaidya, a Minister in the Thai Prime Minister's Office, urgently warned: "Our neighbours are coming over the border and taking the virus back. This is not just a health issue, it's a social issue. We are fighting a lot of ignorance and vested interests."[7]

However, if the deadly combination of intravenous drug-use and the international sex trade first caused HIV/AIDS to make such a rapid impact in Burma, there are also a number of equally salient factors inside Burma that have ensured its continuing spread. Pre-eminent of these are the lack of relevant health information, the shortage of condoms and blood-testing equipment, unhygienic injecting practices, frequent job migration by miners, truckers, fishermen and other occupational groups, and, finally, a cultural environment which makes AIDS a difficult issue to confront. Equally important, it was largely among ethnic minority or other disadvantaged peoples in remote border regions that the AIDS epidemic first developed. Central government authorities were quite incapable of identifying the issue of AIDS or responding effectively in these marginalized and neglected areas. There were no democratic institutions or local systems of health management. Indeed, there appeared to be no cognizance at all that health issues among minority peoples, many of whom were living in or around war zones, have a direct impact on the well-being of the nation as a whole.

Far too belatedly, the SLORC government has begun to respond. The first case of HIV-infection was identified in Burma in 1988. But when the scale of the crisis was finally confirmed by the results of the first sero-sentinel surveillances during 1992-93, according to one international specialist in the sociology of health behaviour, it was "already present at high epidemic levels throughout geographically disparate parts of the country".[8]

The reliability and ethics regarding confidentiality of some of these first surveys have since been questioned by senior health practitioners; it is believed, for example, that, amongst high risk groups, doctors selected individuals for testing in certain parts of the country whom they suspected were already HIV-infected rather than surveying representative cross-samples of particular social groups. The results, nevertheless, demonstrated the high incidence of HIV. The surveys found that 62.8 per cent of all intravenous drug users tested nationally were HIV-positive, but in some areas the rate was even higher: over 90 per cent in the Kachin State and over 80 per cent in Mandalay tested HIV-positive.[9] Other social groupings also showed significant rates of HIV-infection. For example, in the busy border-trading town of Tachilek, 12 per cent of pregnant women tested positive, while in the port-town of Kawthaung, also on the Thai border, the rate among pregnant women was 6 per cent. In this latter town, around

20 per cent of males with other sexually-transmitted diseases also proved positive.[10]

Such alarming findings finally brought an important shift in the public attitudes of the government to the crisis. After several years of official denial that there was any risk of HIV-infection in Burma (until 1991, cartoons in the state-controlled media depicted AIDS as a "foreigners' disease"[11]), a number of AIDS-awareness and prevention campaigns were initiated, with various UN agencies playing an important supporting role. A national AIDS committee had, in fact, been established under the Minister of Health in 1989, but it took until 1991-1992 for the Ministry to formulate its first National AIDS Control and Prevention Plan. With financial backing from the UNDP and the WHO, a number of projects were agreed, including the introduction of the sero-sentinel surveys, blood screening and counselling. Since this time, the UNDCP has also commissioned its first studies on the close link between intravenous drug use and the spread of HIV-infection in Burma, while UNICEF has helped develop a national project on the "Control of HIV/AIDS through Reproductive Health" in conjunction with the Ministry of Health and the Ministry's three chosen NGOs: the MRC, MMCWA and MMA. By mid-1995, this programme was underway in 25 townships especially chosen for their high risk of HIV-infection.

In another important change of policy, despite initial reluctance by the SLORC, several of the first international NGOs to be allowed to return to Burma have been permitted to start AIDS-awareness programmes in selected government-controlled regions of the country. In the past two years, Médicins du Monde has worked at drug rehabilitation centres and sponsored workshops for trainers on AIDS; World Vision has set up an educational programme in AIDS-awareness in partnership with the MMA in the border-town of Kawthaung; and the Association Francois-Xavier Bagnoud has developed a project to assist the social reintegration of former Burmese prostitutes, including those who are HIV-positive. Such collaboration between independent foreign aid organizations in Burma and government authorities would have been unthinkable just a few years ago.

At the national level, too, the SLORC has also given apparent priority to disseminating information on the health risks of HIV/AIDS. By the end of 1995, an estimated 80 per cent of public doctors and medical officers were reported to have undergone basic training in AIDS prevention and diagnosis. Attempts have also been made to get the same message over to the general public. AIDS-awareness posters are publicly displayed in most urban areas today. In broaching this subject, some important cultural taboos have had to be tackled. For example, in 1991 UNICEF produced a one-hour film for Burmese television entitled "Poisonous Love", in which a young man contracts HIV from a prostitute and then infects his wife and, possibly, newborn child. However, it reportedly took UNICEF a further year to persuade the authorities to broadcast the film, since government censors were adamant that a scene showing condoms was offensive in a Buddhist country and must therefore be cut. Eventually, a direct appeal to Lieutenant-General Khin Nyunt, the SLORC Secretary-One, resulted in permission being granted. "Khin Nyunt's wife is a physician, thank goodness," one Western health worker told the *New York Times*. "Otherwise, it might never have gotten on the air."[12]

Since this time, although conservative in language, the dangers of AIDS and possible methods of transmission have been reported quite often in the state-controlled media. Equally important, such commentaries generally reflect the realities of Burmese custom and health in a manner which is very new. Reported the *New Light of Myanmar* on 20 October 1994: "Because only 17 per cent of the population has access to contraceptives, sexually active men and women are at risk, particularly if they have different sexual partners over time."

Yet despite these first moments of health *glasnost*, SLORC officials have remained exceedingly sensitive to international criticism of their handling of the AIDS crisis. Adverse comments in the foreign media have met with stinging rebuttals. For example, when the *Bangkok Post* of 16 September 1994 painted a grim picture of the plight of AIDS patients in the Contagious Diseases Hospital in Rangoon, the response was immediate. Both Vice-Admiral Than Nyunt, the Minister of Health, and Dr Hla Myint, Director-General of the Department of Health, launched strong defences of the government's work in the *New Light of Myanmar*, accusing the international press of "exaggerating for political purposes".[13]

Government doctors, too, have expressed frustration at the opprobrium which they feel has been attached to their work because of international rejection of the SLORC. Although usually privately expressed, such views reached a broader audience during an AIDS conference in Chiang Mai, Thailand, in 1995 which the SLORC allowed a Burmese medical delegation to attend. Matters came to a head when John Dwyer, an Australian immunologist, warned that the Burmese government was making serious mistakes in its response to the epidemic. In reply, Dr Bo Kywe, Deputy Director of Burma's National AIDS Programme, told a press conference that Dwyer was "absolutely incorrect": "People like him who are walking on the international stage have to highlight some points; a lot of people are walking in this way."[14] Dr Kywe, however, did acknowledge that AIDS was not under control in Burma: "We won't be either optimistic or pessimistic, but we are trying to do our best."[15]

The polarity of views expressed in such exchanges only serves to highlight the difficulties in finding common ground to address health issues in a country as riven by political conflict as Burma. Without the institutions of democratic and accountable government, even the fundamental health issue of AIDS can become a deeply political question. As a result, both Burmese opposition groups and many international NGOs have called for a moratorium on the resumption of any international assistance to Burma that is granted in collaboration with the SLORC government until political reform and unrestricted access to the community are both guaranteed (see Chapter 9). However, not all health workers are convinced that international boycotts and pressure on the SLORC are the best solution for such a global emergency as AIDS. "One of the critical problems facing Burma now is its political isolation," argued Daniel Tarantola, AIDS programme director of the Francois-Xavier Bagnoud Centre for Health and Human Rights at the Harvard School of Public Health. "By applying political pressure on the few, the world is penalising the many."[16]

The critical question, then, is whether the health programmes now being instituted under the SLORC will halt the continuing spread of the disease. Certainly, recent random surveys by different health workers have indicated a high public awareness in government-controlled areas of the existence of AIDS, although not necessarily of every aspect of its transmission.

However, despite the recent changes, there remain vast geographical areas and sectors of society where any impact has been minimal. Many health workers fear that for many citizens, it is already a case of "too little, too late". Another problem is that the belated national profile given to the dangers of HIV-infection is in no way matched by the availability of treatment. Outside the main towns and cities, blood screening is still minimal. According to both government and WHO officials, even the proportion of blood samples screened nationally can "not be verified".[17] Indeed, if predictions are correct, as the numbers of AIDS sufferers begin to rise over the next decade, the crisis in HIV/AIDS will be moving from one of "awareness and prevention" programmes to the treatment and human rights' protection of patients. Already such locally-endemic health problems as tuberculosis, drug addiction, hepatitis and malnutrition are believed to take several years off the average life expectancy of HIV-infected persons in Burma when compared with sufferers in the West. Experience in border areas of northern Thailand has also warned that the lives of babies born to HIV-infected mothers are likely to be especially at risk.

In turn, the medical problems of future generations of AIDS sufferers raise a plethora of issues over their rights to treatment, privacy and health information. Those likely to be most affected are the younger generation, with worrying implications for families where the main breadwinners are stricken by illness, and ethnic minority communities in border regions where the disease may already be endemic. In particular, hill peoples such as the Akha in the southern Shan State, where heroin addiction is rife and many of whose young women have worked as prostitutes in Thailand, stand in danger of decimation.

For any of these problems to be addressed, one unifying factor will be restoration of the right to freedom of expression and opinion. Freedom of expression is the only universal guarantee by which the quality of research can be improved and the rights of local communities to information and participation in health issues can be protected. But as UNICEF has warned, "No comprehensive national education and communication programme yet exists."[18]

At the same time, it is important to note that, since 1992, the SLORC and Ministry of Health have allowed a growing number of foreign specialists to work on this issue. Those given permission to enter Burma, however, have swiftly become aware of the enormous difficulties in establishing any reliable information or data. According to Doug Porter, who conducted research in 1994 supported by the

UNDP, Rangoon Institute of Economics and the Australian National University:

> Before undertaking the research, none of the team was sanguine about the difficulties to be encountered, but none anticipated the realities. Field research activities were in practice severely restricted and abbreviated in terms of their overall duration; the localities visited (e.g. the central Wa region was not visited); representativeness (e.g., hill-top Wa villages were not accessed); and in terms of the veracity of information gathered ... . Furthermore, planned research activities often had to give way to the exigencies of military and security interests in the area, including everyday military surveillance, itinerant banditry, *Tatmadaw* operational activities, and instability in some of the militia-controlled areas.[19]

Thus, as international experience the world over has suggested, while both political and social conditions remain unchanged, there is unlikely to be much substantive impact on the spread of HIV/AIDS — especially on the margins of society. In Burma, the rapid migration of many workers remains one major factor.[20] But perhaps the most difficult to tackle remains the increasing practice of heroin abuse, which has long been a serious, though much neglected, health problem in its own right.

As always in Burma, there is a considerable gulf between official descriptions of the narcotics trade and the grim reality itself. Burma is a State Party to both the 1961 Single Convention on Narcotics Drugs and the 1988 UN Convention against Illicit Traffic in Narcotic Drugs and Psychotropic Substances. In 1993, the SLORC also promulgated a new Narcotics Drugs and Psychotropic Substances Law to replace 1974 legislation from the BSPP era and to further prohibit all drug use, possession or trafficking with the threat of long jail terms. At the same time, since 1989 the SLORC has entered Burma into programmes of sub-regional co-operation, supported by the UNDCP, with China, Thailand, Laos, Cambodia and Vietnam, as well as through bilateral agreements with both India and Bangladesh. Reflecting these programmes, official government reports now frequently use the language of development and crop-substitution. Nevertheless, senior SLORC officers and the state-controlled media continue to depict Burma's narcotics problem in the most propagandist terms as essentially being a "war" of interdiction, always being waged successfully by the *Tatmadaw*. "Which country in the world has sacrificed the lives of over 190 soldiers with an additional 350 wounded in the combat against drug traffickers in a matter of only four weeks?" the SLORC Foreign Minister, U Ohn Gyaw, asked the UN General Assembly on 11 October 1994.

In such a highly censored environment, the scale of Burma's drugs problem is never publicly revealed. For decades, the illicit opium trade within the country has remained hidden by secrecy and danger; the twin problems of armed opposition and narcotics are inextricably linked. But while Burma's political deadlock continues, the main elements in the trade remain impervious to change: the impoverished hill farmers who grow the opium poppies; the armed opposition groups, local militia and traders who transport the raw opium and refine it into heroin; the corruption and indifference of government officials; and, finally, the international syndicates who transport the finished product into the world markets. Indeed, according to the US State Department, despite the spread of cease-fires in the war zones, Burma's annual opium harvest has more than doubled since the SLORC assumed power in 1988 to over 2,000 tons per annum.[21] Some 60 per cent of the heroin for sale on the streets of the USA today is believed to originate from Burma.[22]

However, while world attention continues to focus on the misleading and elusive search for a few "Mr Bigs" who are alleged to control the trade, the alarming health consequences for the Burmese peoples have been dangerously overlooked. There has long been a simplistic tradition of blaming the trade on different political protagonists in Burma — from the Burmese government, Communist Party of Burma or Chinese Kuomintang remnants to local ethnic minority or militia leaders such as Lo Hsing-han and Khun Sa.[23] For their part, SLORC officials in the present day continue to claim the trade is a heritage of the colonial era under the British, who left Burma back in 1948.[24]

Fatal Silence?

The reality is that the international narcotics trade has long spawned its own corruption, and such arguments do little to address the health impact of narcotics on local inhabitants. In the 1980s, for example, Burma's Shan State was the scene of a grave but indiscriminate abuse of health rights when, largely unreported, over 60,000 acres of highland forest and dozens of ethnic minority villages were sprayed from the air by the Burmese air force with the US-supplied 2,4-D, a compound used in the production of Agent Orange, without any warning to the local people. Food and water supplies were contaminated, and a variety of health disorders were reported by villagers who migrated towards the Thai border. In fact, little of the wealth associated with the narcotics trade ever reaches the impoverished inhabitants of north-east Burma, except for a small class of entrepreneurs who have flourished under the SLORC's "open-door" economic policy. Indeed, during the crop-spraying period, opium production actually went up; for impoverished hill-farmers there is simply no other cash crop.[25]

After years of conflict, the plight of many communities in the main poppy-growing areas is now desperate, and there has been an upsurge in intravenous drug use over the past decade as more and more opium is locally refined into heroin. This changing pattern of drug abuse has coincided with the advent of HIV/AIDS, with disastrous consequences. Whether through undiagnosed cases of AIDS, drug overdoses, meningitis, tuberculosis, septicaemia, hepatitis or other related health problems, the few qualified practitioners still working in the area have reported an alarming loss of life. In many areas, community leaders privately say that it is hard to find a single family without at least one addict.

So alarmed was one armed opposition group, the Kachin Independence Organization, by the explosion in drug abuse in the late 1980s (and by the rise in what it correctly predicted to be AIDS) that it passed its own legislation and began a drug eradication programme of its own. This campaign began in horrifying circumstances. Having recorded 328 drug-related deaths in the jade mining region of Hpakhan between November 1989 and April 1990, the KIO publicly executed 54 alleged drug dealers and offenders in August 1990 in scenes which were videotaped and widely circulated. "We firmly believe we have no other alternative than the use of the death penalty in individual cases of continued violation of our drug laws," explained a KIO official at one international seminar.[26]

From its initial strongholds in the Shan and Kachin States, the practice of intravenous drug use has now spread across the country and can be found in both Mandalay and Rangoon. Former inmates, for example, claim that heroin is easily available in prisons, where many drug offenders end up at some stage.[27] It also remains particularly cheap and widely available in the jade mining regions of the Kachin State and the ruby mines of the Shan State. From such local centres, HIV/AIDS has continued to spread amongst intravenous drug users. This was belatedly confirmed by the 1992 sero-sentinel surveillance tests in which 62.8 per cent of all IDUs tested nationally were HIV-positive, one of the highest sectoral figures ever recorded in the world. By the following March, this figure had grown to 74.3 per cent.[28]

Although occasionally alluded to in the country's new business press, none of these serious health issues is ever reflected in the state-controlled media. There are undoubtedly government officials, just as there are opposition groups, who are anxious to begin effective drug eradication and rehabilitation programmes. In most major towns, for example, government-sponsored drug treatment programmes have long existed. In the last four years, the UNDCP has also been allowed to initiate pilot crop-substitution programmes in the Shan State. But without political reform, there remain many obstacles in the way to taking the kind of concerted actions that are required; sheer survival and political expediency still predominate. Simply too much money is being made, and not just by corrupt officials or armed opposition groups (notably the UWSP and MTA of Khun Sa) which control much of the poppy-growing region and opium trade. It is one of the most open secrets in Burma today that much of the large profit made through narcotics is laundered through official trade and other new business projects that are currently under way in Mandalay, Rangoon and the other main conurbations.

Faced with this aid vacuum, many community groups, especially those based around Christian churches and Buddhist monasteries, have instituted their own narcotics and AIDS awareness programmes in the towns. Several armed opposition groups also publicly advocate anti-narcotics policies. US Drug Enforcement Agency officials, for example, have privately admitted the success of the KIO in decreasing poppy cultivation in its operational areas, while the USWP has repeatedly called for direct international assistance which bypasses the SLORC.[29] This is a step, however, few international health or development agencies are prepared to countenance for fear of jeopardizing their relations with Rangoon and the SLORC. The fact remains that, until political reform and stability are ensured, many of the most vulnerable or affected groups will remain beyond effective outreach.

As a result, the drug culture in Burma today continues to survive against a backdrop of ignorance and lack of information. Even the particular HIV/AIDS explosion that occurred in Burma can be put down to very ill-informed behaviour about health risks. For example, intravenous drug users commonly visit "shooting galleries" where dealers inject groups of addicts using unsterilized, self-made equipment — such as needles attached to eye-droppers or polythene tubes — that is repeatedly used. In these areas, many quacks and even qualified doctors also give repeat, unhygienic injections. International AIDS specialists are thus convinced that such unsanitary practices, combined with the already high prevalence of the disease among a mobile social group, account for the extraordinarily fast spread of HIV-infection in north-east Burma. For example, one sample survey of 73 drug addicts from Hpakhan in the Kachin State found that 91 per cent were HIV-positive, of whom 47 per cent had used drugs "for six months or less" and only 16 per cent had been using drugs "for more than two years". Moreover, although most were sexually active, 80 per cent had never heard of condoms.[30]

Built upon such bedrocks of ignorance, it is difficult to see how existing legislation or programmes can cope with the twin perils of drug abuse and AIDS. Even the total drug output in Burma is the subject of controversy. Although producing no alternative figures, SLORC officials have consistently accused Western anti-narcotics agencies of exaggerating Burma's opium harvest, a claim some armed opposition groups would support. But even the widely quoted figure of over 2,000 tons per annum in the West is largely based upon satellite imagery and sample field-surveys, and it must therefore be seen, at best, as a guesstimate.

Similarly, there are no reliable estimates for the number of drug addicts in Burma today. Over 50,000 addicts have officially registered since rehabilitation programmes began at public drug treatment centres in 1974, but the true number of addicts must be considerably higher. The KIO estimates that there are 33,500 opium and heroin addicts in the Kachin State alone.[31]

Adding to these uncertainties, there are also serious problems with the drug treatment that is available in Burma, as well as the relevant legislation. Many medical practitioners believe that, given the lack of resources, drug treatment centres are well-organized and provide one of the best public services in the country. However, addicts commonly relapse after treatment; centres are often far from patients' homes; and current legislation, which requires addicts to register voluntarily or face jail terms of up to five years, simply forces many to go underground. Equally important, while the government has switched from a policy of silence on contraception to one of advocating condom use in order to prevent the sexual transmission of AIDS, sweeping changes are still needed to pharmaceutical legislation which currently outlaws the non-medical possession of syringes and needles.

In conclusion, given this terrible background of AIDS and drug abuse, many people in Burma are questioning why the SLORC government is taking no effective action against the country's enormous trade in illicit opium. Exactly the same question is being asked among international anti-narcotics agencies and, as a sign of such concerns, in November 1995 President Clinton signed a Presidential Decision Directive withholding US aid, including through the International Monetary Fund and World Bank, from countries such as Burma where US officials do not believe governments are "co-operating" to stop the flow of heroin.[32]

Less than two months later, the SLORC agreed a cease-fire with the 15,000-strong MTA of Khun Sa, which had previously been denounced in the state-controlled media as the main trafficking force. Government troops were allowed to enter MTA positions, and two doctors were sent from Rangoon to Khun Sa's headquarters at Homong to care for him. United States officials were outraged: already under indictment in the US for heroin trafficking, a two million US dollar reward was offered for information leading to his capture.

Nevertheless, with the MTA truce, the central Burmese government has achieved its first apparent peace in north-east Burma in decades. Cease-fires have also been sustained since 1989 with the other key armed ethnic opposition forces involved in the narcotics trade, notably the UWSP and Myanmar National Defence Alliance Army, which control the prize poppy fields in the Wa and Kokang sub-states respectively. The KIO, too, which agreed a cease-fire in 1994, continues its own eradication and rehabilitation programmes.

On the surface, then, it appears an opportune time to address the underlying economic and political issues that have long underpinned ethnic conflict and the opium trade. No side believes political and development solutions will be either quick or easy, but there has never been a better moment to try.

At the moment, however, the drugs trade still continues in conditions of great secrecy and doubt about the government's intentions. For while the SLORC has reportedly given orders to Khun Sa's supporters to stop heroin refining in MTA areas along the Thai border, over the past year the *Tatmadaw* has quietly taken control of the important drugs-trafficking town of Mongko on the Chinese border after clashes between rival Kokangese cease-fire militia. Here, opposition sources in the drugs trade estimate that 10 per cent of all heroin-refining in the Shan State takes place. Indeed, recent travellers report poppy cultivation has been flourishing throughout north-east Burma this year, with good weather conditions and little sign of government interdiction.

Health workers and community groups, nevertheless, are still quietly pressing for substantive action. One recent survey by local health workers of AIDS and narcotics abuse in north-east Burma uncovered rates of over 40 per cent addiction in some villages, where deaths are reported to be occurring nearly every day. According to a private appeal that was circulated to international donors:

> The younger generation, in particular, is in danger
> of near extermination if something is not done to
> control a wider spread of AIDS. It is with this hope
> that we make an appeal to humanitarian groups eve-
> rywhere all over the world.

NOTES

[1] See e.g., AFP, 21 Sept. 1995; UNICEF, *Children and Women in Myanmar*

(see Chapter 2, note 13), 42.

[2] ARTICLE 19, *State of Fear* (see Chapter 1, note 4), 12.

[3] Reuters, 1 June 1994, 25 Feb. 1995.

[4] *Bangkok Post*, 26 Feb. 1995.

[5] See e.g., Smith, *Ethnic Groups in Burma* (see Chapter 6, note 2), 114; Human Rights Watch/Asia, *A Modern Form of Slavery: Trafficking of Burmese Women and Girls into Brothels in Thailand* (New York: 1993), 14.

[6] UNICEF, note 1 above, at 42.

[7] *Burma Alert*, June 1991.

[8] G V Stimson PhD, *Drug Injecting and the Spread of HIV Infection in South-East Asia* (conference paper, to be published in proceedings of 2nd AIDS IMPACT Conference, Brighton, UK, July 1994), 12.

[9] Source: Department of Health, Rangoon.

[10] Ibid.

[11] See e.g., *Working People's Daily*, 30 July 1991.

[12] *New York Times*, 11 March 1994.

[13] *New Light of Myanmar*, 27 Sept. and 11 Oct. 1994. Although few people in Burma have access to international newspapers such as the *Bangkok Post*, these reports are often picked up and rebroadcast in the Burmese language by other media in the region, including Voice of America (VOA) and the BBC. The BBC has also run its own series of Burmese-language programmes on AIDS, which proved popular in the country. Since August 1995, however, both the BBC and VOA have been intermittently jammed by the Burmese authorities for the first time ever, apparently to prevent political interviews and independent news being heard following the release of Aung San Suu Kyi.

[14] *The Nation* (Bangkok), 21 Sept. 1995.

[15] Ibid.

[16] Reuters, 30 July 1993.

[17] Min Thwe and Bo Kywe, National AIDS Programme, D J Goodwin, (WHO), *HIV Surveillance in Myanmar, 1985-95* (Conference paper, III International Conference on AIDS in Asia and the Pacific, Chiang Mai, Sept. 1995), 4.

[18] UNICEF, note 1 above, at 42.

[19] Porter, *Wheeling and Dealing* (see Chapter 4, note 18), 93.

[20] For example, when World Vision conducted research to begin its AIDS programme in Kawthaung, 31 commercial sex workers were interviewed; two years later, all such workers had disappeared by either moving or going "underground"; see, World Vision, *Report on Review of the AIDS Awareness, Education and Prevention Project in Kawthaung* (MMA and World Vision, Rangoon: May 1995), 12. For other social factors, see also, Southeast Asian Information Network, *Out of Control: The HIV/AIDS Epidemic in Burma* (Chiang Mai: 1995), 6-12.

[21] *The Nation* (Bangkok), 13 March 1992; US General Accounting Office, *Drug Control: US Heroin Program Encounters Many Obstacles in Southeast Asia* (Washington: 1996), 3.

[22] US Department of State, *International Narcotics Control Strategy Report* (Washington: March 1996).

[23] Smith, *Burma: Insurgency and the Politics of Ethnicity* (see Chapter 6, note 1), 314-315.

[24] *Drugs Suppression in Myanmar: Tatmadaw Role in Combating the Scourge of Illicit Drugs* (mimeograph, Rangoon: Ministry of Information, July 1996), 1. For a more detailed analysis, see, *The Heroin Wars* (Channel 4 TV, UK, July 1996).

[25] For an investigation, see, US General Accounting Office, *Drug Control: Enforcement Efforts in Burma are not Effective* (Washington: 1989).

[26] Col. Zau Seng, *Establishing Anti-Drug Policies in a Liberated Zone of Burma* (Statement of KIO to International Symposium: Illicit Drugs and Global Geopolitics, Paris: Dec. 1992), 7.

[27] According to one survey, 70 per cent of 500 prisoners in Lashio jail were convicted under narcotics legislation, while 790 of the 4,000 prisoners in Mandalay jail were drug offenders, some 70 per cent of whom were IDUs; see, *HIV Infection and Injecting Drug Use in the Union of Myanmar: A report to the United Nations International Drug Control Programme by Professor Gerry V Stimson* (Final Report, 9 Feb. 1994), 16-17. There is also concern over the health treatment of drug offenders in prison, including those who are HIV-positive. In many prison hospitals (which are often regarded as good places to be admitted from a cell), drug offenders constitute a large percentage of the patients, including around 40 per cent in Mandalay. However former prisoners report that some doctors have, in the past, often carried out multiple injections on prisoners by repeatedly using just one needle without out sterilization.

28 Ibid., at 4-6.

29 See e.g., Ta Saw Lu, *The Bondage of Opium: The Agony of the Wa People* (UWSP Foreign Affairs Department: 1993).

30 Stimson, note 27 above, at 8, 11.

31 Col. Zau Seng, note 26 above, at 9.

32 AP, 18 Dec. 1995. As one of the world's main sufferers, the US government faces particular problems in combating the heroin trade. All anti-narcotics and development aid to Burma was suspended in 1988 in protest at the SLORC's assumption of power. Since this time, successive administrations have refused to resume any eradication assistance to Burma until there is evidence of human rights reform, which restores political rights to the people. The US General Accounting Office recently reaffirmed: "Because of the complex Burmese political environment, US assistance is unlikely to be effective until the Burmese government demonstrates improvement in its democracy and human rights policies and proves its legitimacy to ethnic minority groups in opium producing areas." See, US General Accounting Office, note 21 above, at 2-3.

Chapter 8

WOMEN AND HEALTH

Despite their respected role in society, women from all ethnic groups in Burma have become extremely vulnerable to the devastating impact of the country's long-running social and political malaise. This is not always apparent to foreign visitors. Women in Burma are visibly active in a great variety of public affairs, especially in commerce, education, health and agriculture. Yet the prominence of Daw Aung San Suu Kyi as a national leader is very much an exception in the male-dominated world of Burmese politics. Gender discrimination severely restricts the right of women to express their legitimate interests in social and political affairs. Although constituting an estimated 40 per cent of the workforce, few women have ever been allowed to rise to top government positions.[1] As a result, the particular health and discrimination problems which many women suffer daily are often overlooked.

In the past few years, a number of international agencies have uncovered evidence of discrimination against women and neglect of their health, but their findings have never been publicly accepted by the Burmese government. Much of this evidence has come from UNICEF and foreign NGOs working with refugee populations along Burma's borders. Although a signatory to the 1952 UN Convention on the Political Rights of Women, Burma has not ratified the 1981 Convention on the Elimination of All Forms of Discrimination Against Women, nor does it have any official agency to advance or protect the status of women.

Under the SLORC, all reports of health or human rights abuses against women continue to be rejected by military spokesmen in blanket fashion. In October 1995, for example, the SLORC responded to the UN Special Rapporteur to Myanmar, who had provided a summary of serious human rights violations against women, by citing the existence of "equal rights" and five key laws which, it argued, would prevent any such abuses occurring: the Suppression of Prostitution Act (1949), the Myanmar Buddhist Women's Special Marriage and Succession Act (1954), the Myanmar Maternal and Child Welfare

Association Law, the Nursing and Maternity Law, and the Penal Code. Claimed the SLORC:

> Women in Myanmar are not only protected by such laws and provisions, they are also protected by Myanmar traditions and customs, as well as customary law, religious beliefs and practices. Women's rights constitute human rights and Myanmar women fully enjoy fundamental rights.[2]

Contradicting such assertions is the evidence of a disturbing pattern of grave human rights abuses and humanitarian neglect throughout Burma since 1988, in which women have often been particular victims. Many of the most serious allegations, including summary arrest, rape or extrajudicial execution, concern violations committed by government soldiers on military operations in ethnic minority regions of the country, where military officers have extraordinary powers of arrest and command.[3]

Another grievance in many areas has been the forcible conscription of women, including girls, pregnant women and the elderly, into compulsory labour duties on government construction projects or even as porters in the war zones. Such "forced labour", as practised in Burma, is also a human rights violation against men or in any other context[4], but the conscription of women additionally contravenes Article 11 of the ILO Convention No. 29 Concerning Forced or Compulsory Labour, ratified by Burma in 1955, which confines compulsory labour to "able-bodied" males aged between 18 and 45. In Burma, however, massive numbers of women have been forced to work on such projects in the past few years. This has major health and humanitarian implications for the whole of Burmese society, since not only does forced labour in itself have an extremely detrimental impact on health, but it is in the course of forced labour duties that many of the worst human rights violations against women, including rape and threats to life, have been committed. In 1991, for example, two Karen high school girls, Naw Aye Hla, aged 17, and Ne Law Win, aged 16, died after they had been conscripted as porters and compelled to walk through a minefield in the hills near Papun.[5] More recently, the underground Burmese Women's Union, which was formed in 1995 by democracy activists in the Thai border region, presented a 30-page dossier of women's sufferings during forced labour to the UN Fourth World Conference on Women in Beijing. "Sometimes we didn't go because we were tired, but they came at night and dragged us from our house," one woman complained. "My children were screaming and crying, but I just had to leave them there."[6]

Reports of gross human rights violations such as these, together with the detention of 1991 Nobel Peace prize winner Aung San Suu Kyi, have attracted most international concern since the SLORC came to power. They have also focused attention on the important role of women in the democracy movement. Suu Kyi herself was eventually released in July 1995 after six years under house arrest without trial, but many other women have also been detained over the past seven years. Prominent among women political prisoners still held today are the writer, Daw San San Nwe, her daughter, Ma Myat Mo Mo Tun, and Dr Ma Thida. Like Dr Khin Zaw Win, San San Nwe and her daughter were accused in 1994 of anti-government activities and of sending "fabricated news" to the UN Special Rapporteur to Myanmar. They received ten and seven year sentences respectively, while Ma Thida, who is serving a 20-year sentence, was arrested with the MP-elect, Dr Aung Khin Sint, in a clamp-down on NLD supporters the previous year (see Chapter 6.3).

Such ill-treatment of women — whether through forced labour, forced relocations or imprisonment — is only indicative of a greater neglect that has developed at the heart of Burmese society in which the basic health and human rights of women have long been denied. Every day women in Burma suffer ill health or die from conditions that should be preventable. Yet, such issues receive little or no publicity at all.

As with the health system overall, the general standards of health care available to women are extremely variable, depending much on class, wealth and the region of the country. But, at a time of deep social upheaval, many health workers believe that large numbers of women bear a "double burden" which is particularly injurious to their health, as both workers and the main carers for their families. Such hardships are most acute in ethnic minority regions where constant relocations and the heavy loss of men in fighting has left many women bringing up families alone. In just one border region of the eastern

Shan State, for example, the UWSP, which agreed a cease-fire with the SLORC in 1989, claims that over 12,000 Wa soldiers were killed and many more disabled in 22 years of armed conflict, leaving innumerable widows and orphans without support in an area which remains beyond the reach of most outside agencies.[7]

Women also suffer considerable hardship, including poverty and poor access to health care, in many of the relocation sites and satellite new towns which the SLORC has built across Burma (see Chapter 6.2.). In 1992 one UNICEF consultant warned:

> The forced displacement of an already vulnerable group of low-income population, who have suffered from chronic poverty, to an area with extremely poor sanitation and living conditions with little or no job opportunities gives rise to a sequence of socio-economic problems, such as unemployment, abandoned wives and children, induced abortion, increased exposure to STDs/AIDS and malnutrition, which need to be addressed promptly.[8]

Even where the evidence is obvious to local health workers, there is no effective system of reporting health news and the government authorities have remained slow to react. The poor provision of sanitation and clean water supplies is one such example. Not only are contaminated water and unsanitary conditions major sources for the spread of some of the most prevalent illnesses in Burma, such as hepatitis and intestinal parasitic diseases, but women and children have traditionally performed the burdensome task of collecting the water. According to the government's own figures, by 1990 only 32.1 per cent of the country was estimated to have access to proper sanitation or clean water.[9] Considerable infrastructural problems remain in any rapid upgrading of facilities. However, the SLORC does not appear to consider this a financial priority. Despite the massive sums evidently available for expenditure on the armed forces, in the official "National Programme of Action for the Survival, Protection and Development of Myanmar's Children in the 1990s" the government claimed that any "extension of these services is precariously dependent on the limited support of UNICEF and other agencies".[10]

Poor levels of educational provision also handicap many women. In rural areas, especially, it is girls rather than boys who are kept home from school to perform domestic chores or help with the farming, and this has long been reflected in the lower literacy rates for women in Burma. Government figures generally show a 15 per cent disparity between national literacy rates for men and women, but in ethnic minority areas, where children also have to learn Burmese as a second language, the gap is even wider, with estimates by community leaders of 80 per cent illiteracy among women in some border regions. Indeed, in remote mountain areas, many girls never attend school. But, as a growing body of international evidence has shown, the education of women is often the key to the health of the whole community. According to UNICEF, "investments in women's education" have resulted in a broad array of social breakthroughs in other parts of the developing world, including falls in infant mortality rates, improvements in the general nutritional status of families, increased educational achievement by children and, equally important, higher incomes and productivity in the community.[11]

The basic health problems, then, that women face in Burma today are considerable. Most are attributable to poor living conditions and lack of access to adequate health care or education. Along with other human rights violations, these are issues which, in the long term, can only be solved by social and political reform.

Two further issues of particular relevance to women, however, require immediate action: the provision of essential reproductive health information and a halt to the continuing traffic of Burmese women into prostitution, where they are especially vulnerable to HIV-infection and the many other dangers of the sex trade.

Reproductive health is one of the least acknowledged health issues in Burma, but as UNICEF recently warned: "The paucity of information on women's reproductive health in Myanmar is in itself an indication that many of their needs are unrecognized."[12] The most obvious indicator of such neglect is Burma's estimated maternal mortality rate of 140 per 100,000 live births, which is the third highest in the East Asia and Pacific region.[13] However even this high figure (which the government acknowledges) is based only upon hospital statistics and is thus likely to be an underestimate. There are wide regional disparities in Burma and no reliable data at all on maternal mortality within the home, where an estimated 80 per cent of all births take place.[14]

Many of these deaths are happening in conditions of great secrecy and silence. Yet, few doctors in Burma have any doubts about the causes of such a high maternal mortality rate, which they attribute to lack of access to reproductive health information, including on contraception and birth spacing programmes, as well as the illegality of abortions. Since abortion is illegal in Burma, doctors often attribute maternal deaths caused by botched abortions to other medical causes — sometimes to spare the women's families public embarrassment but, more often, simply to avoid investigations or extra work. Such caution is pervasive. However, 50 per cent of all maternal deaths are estimated to result directly from illicit abortions that might have been avoided altogether if reproductive health information and affordable contraception had been available. UNICEF, for example, estimated in 1992 that 58 women were dying every week from illegal abortions.[15]

The evidence is stark. Health workers across the country privately report that, every day, women of childbearing age resort to various methods of abortion, ranging from the use of indigenous medicines to induce bleeding to illegal operations carried out by private doctors, or the desperate use of quacks who use sticks and other crude implements to abort foetuses for as little as 200 kyats (US$ 2). Every doctor and midwife in Burma can tell of illicit abortions that have gone terribly wrong, resulting in the deaths of young and frightened mothers. The full scale of such incidents, however, is never officially reported by the public health authorities due to a conspiracy of silence which all parties prefer to maintain until there is a fundamental change in public attitudes and law.

Many other fatalities also result from causes which would be preventable with adequate access for women to health information. These include common complaints that are aggravated by pregnancy, such as malaria, hepatitis and malnutrition. For example, over 60 per cent of pregnant women in Burma — or 700,000 women annually — are estimated to suffer from iron deficiency anaemia, while iodine and other nutritional deficiencies are equally prevalent in many areas of the country.[16] Equally important, many doctors believe that the poor nutritional status of mothers is responsible for the high levels of preterm or low birth weight deliveries in Burma and, possibly, for growth-retarded or brain-damaged babies, leaving yet another legacy of public health care problems for future generations to address.

Nonetheless, while the subject of abortion largely remains taboo, official attitudes are belatedly beginning to change on the question of reproductive health information, largely in response to the pandemic spread of AIDS. Under the influence of various UN agencies, the SLORC government is slowly beginning to shift from a pro-natalist policy and accept that the public has a right to information about contraception and reproductive health. For the moment, however, reproductive health education is not available on a country-wide basis within the public health system, and access to contraception remains scarce. Since 1991, birth spacing programmes have been carried out in only 31 townships with the support of UN agencies and the Family Planning International Assistance.

It is now also accepted by both the Health Ministry and international agencies that women from Burma are especially vulnerable to HIV-infection for a variety of reasons, including unprotected sexual intercourse with infected male partners, unhygienic injections and the frequent need for blood transfusions after childbirth because of anaemia or poor perinatal care, and the large numbers of women working as prostitutes in Thailand or Burma. Indeed, health officials estimate that women constitute at least a third of all cases of HIV-infection in Burma (or over 175,000 individuals), and this high incidence among women is also indicated in all the sero-sentinel survey data collected since 1992.[17] As a result, in 1993 a project for the "Control of HIV/AIDS through Reproductive Health" was begun in six townships in a partnership between the Ministry of Health, UNICEF and the SLORC's preferred NGOs — the MRC, MMCWA and MMA — with additional support from the WHO, UNDP and UN Population Fund (UNPFA). These education programmes focus on high-risk young women and men and had spread to 25 townships by 1995, with the aim of reaching 103 of Burma's 319 townships by the end of the century. At the same time, new emphasis is being given to better reproductive health training for midwives, auxiliary nurses and community volunteers who, it is intended, will act as the next generation of educators.

Yet, there still remains a massive task ahead. With widespread restrictions still imposed on the media, freedom of expression and the right to community participation, many health workers doubt how effectively these efforts will reach the most vulnerable and needy members of society. Since 1988, the official contraception prevalence rate is only estimated to have risen from 13 per cent of the female population of reproductive age to between 17 and 22 per cent, still considerably short of the goal set by the Health Ministry and UNPFA of 30 per cent by 1997.[18]

For the moment, the reality is that the majority of Burmese women remain extremely under-informed on reproductive health matters, and such information is not supplied in any systematic way in the state-controlled media. In many areas, superstitious beliefs that can have an adverse affect on women's health remain common. Doctors, for example, complain that, after child delivery, many women will not touch soap for up to a month since they believe it can cause sickness.

Compounding these problems, government health centres are invariably under-funded and under-staffed, while the estimated 8,000 local midwives often have impossibly large areas to serve which can become inaccessible in the rainy season. As a result, although some effort has been made to provide antenatal care in urban areas, an estimated third of all births in Burma take place without the presence of trained medical personnel, and many women prefer to rely on private medicine (of variable quality) for reproductive health matters if they have access to the towns. For the few who can afford it, high quality modern health treatment is available, including sterilization for women (for which official permission is needed) and vasectomies for men (which are illegal). But most women are forced to depend on the private market to purchase contraceptives, where there are considerable concerns about quality control and medical supervision. Four contraceptive methods are generally available in urban areas today: Depo Progesterone injections (which are probably the most popular), contraceptive pills, intra-uterine devices and condoms (which are usually only purchased by men and are unpopular with some married couples since they have traditionally been associated with prostitution).

As Burma's reproductive health programmes expand, such questions as condom use, birth control and other matters related to health rights will inevitably require full public explanation and debate. Already there have been reports of dissension among Muslim communities in the Rakhine State, where the recent availability of Depo

Progesterone injections has led to incorrect rumours, largely spread by men, that the SLORC authorities were attempting to sterilize all Muslim women as a form of social control. In the Rakhine State, as elsewhere in Burma, ethnic population statistics remain a major, although unpublicized, political issue.

Major challenges are also likely to be faced on the issue of condom use to stop the spread of HIV/AIDS and other sexually-transmitted diseases. This issue is closely interlinked with prostitution, yet another of Burma's hidden health issues. In this deeply conservative country, imbued with Buddhist traditions, prostitution remains illegal and is rarely publicly acknowledged. Yet this issue above all demonstrates the close connection between censorship, the vulnerability of uneducated women and the importance of access to essential health information to allow people to make informed choices on matters affecting their health.

The scale of indigenous prostitution in Burma is impossible to calculate. Much of the trade is extremely shadowy and mobile, with many young women (some as young as 12) frequently moving house or directly being brought to clients at night while under the control of different madames and pimps. Some young women are forced to enter prostitution to support their families, while others have taken it up while trying to eke out a living on the streets. However, by all estimates, the number of active commercial sex workers has increased dramatically in response to the social and economic upheavals in Burma since 1988. In major towns, many restaurants and night-clubs are thinly-disguised brothels, while in the mining boom towns of the north-east many small brothels exist openly. Over 100 brothels of varying sizes are operational in the Hpakhan jade-mining area alone, where high rates of HIV-infection have been recorded among intravenous drug users (see Chapter 7). Elsewhere, many commercial sex workers simply move around the country also earning money as traders or working as prostitutes out of roadside tea-shops and restaurants.[19]

Many young prostitutes remain woefully uninformed about the risks they take. Under the 1949 Prostitution Suppression Act, four training schools, with capacity for up to 600 former sex workers, have been set up in Rangoon, Mandalay, Mergui and Kengtung under the Department of Social Welfare.[20] As a result, women attending these schools were chosen for some of the first HIV-testing and AIDS-awareness programmes in Burma. But, as an illustration of the problems to be faced, of 78 residents interviewed in 1994 by UNICEF in one training school, 70 per cent had sexually-transmitted diseases and seven were HIV-positive. Moreover, 98 per cent had no knowledge of AIDS or how it could be prevented.[21]

Doctors in Burma, however, believe that women who work in the Thai sex industry run an even greater risk of exposure to HIV/AIDS and other health dangers. In Thailand, HIV/AIDS and other sexually-transmitted diseases have reached epidemic proportions in the sex industry. Burmese male emigrants who frequent prostitutes in Thailand, especially fishermen and labourers, also carry the HIV virus back to Burma, but this latter population group has not, until recently, been closely identified in public health policy — even though fishermen, at least, should be easy to gain access to. For this reason, most international health education concern has, instead, been focused on women.

The numbers of women and girls from Burma working in prostitution in Thailand is undoubtedly large, with estimates of up to 40,000 at any one time today. Often advertised as AIDS-free but lacking Thai language skills, many are forced to work at the cheapest and most dangerous end of the market, where rates of up to 90 per cent HIV-infection have been recorded. In some brothels a form of debt bondage also exists, and beatings and over 15 deaths have been reported.[22]

Partly in response to international expression of health and human rights concern, in 1993 the Chuan government in Thailand launched a suppression policy against the sex industry but, although there are now fewer brothels, the number of sex workers — whether Thai or immigrant — has not markedly decreased. Young women from Burma still form a substantial proportion of the sex workers in many borderland areas, especially in Chiang Mai and northern Thailand and in the border sea-port of Ranong, opposite Kawthaung.

There are many factors which induce so many women from Burma to work as prostitutes in Thailand. Some have been lured there, while others have been forced. But the one common denominator they share is social deprivation: nearly all come from poor backgrounds and lack educational opportunities or provision. A majority of them are thought to be from ethnic minorities, which constitute some of Burma's most marginalized communities from borderland regions, where women, as a group, are more marginalized still. This is evident in the particularly low literacy rates for women in these areas. For example, a recent survey of nearly 200 young people in one remote district of the Shan State recorded that 72.4 per cent of women were illiterate as against only 24.5 per cent of men; moreover, in poor rural areas female illiteracy reached 86.2 per cent.[23] Concrete data is still lacking on many aspects of the commercial sex trade and many regional disparities are likely. But according to one 1992 investigation for UNICEF, in some communities in the eastern Shan State around 20 per cent of all females aged 15 to 25 were working as prostitutes in Thailand at any one time.[24]

Following a well-reported incident in early 1996, when two groups of female dancers (including one from a *Tatmadaw* officer's family) were tricked into signing up for performance tours to Japan where their hosts tried to force them into prostitution, the SLORC briefly reacted by taking the extreme measure of trying to prevent the departure on their own from Rangoon of any single women holding Burmese passports. However, not only is this a gross infringement on the right of all women to freedom of association and travel, but it merely accelerated the unregulated exodus of women across Burma's other frontiers.

For all such issues to be addressed, it is therefore absolutely vital that matters relating to education, freedom of expression and information and women's health are brought to the fore in public debate and treated as urgent areas requiring social and political reform.

NOTES

[1] In 1991-1992, for example, there were 60,708 women in higher education as compared to 45,948 men. Women teachers also outnumber men by two to one, but few women have been promoted to top posts in the education system; see, M Smith, "Burma (Myanmar)", in World University Service, *Academic Freedom 3: Education and Human Rights* (London: Zed Books, 1995), 105. Many women feel that similar discrimination exists in the health sector, where women are also in the majority if all jobs are included.

[2] UN General Assembly, *Situation of Human Rights in Myanmar* (see Chapter

2, note 21), 30.

[3] See e.g., Amnesty International, *Myanmar: The climate of fear continues, members of ethnic minorities and political prisoners still targeted* (London: 1993), 18-21; Human Rights Watch/Asia, *Burma: Rape, Forced Labour and Religious Persecution* (see Chapter 6, note 40), 6-11; Smith, *Ethnic Groups in Burma* (see Chapter 6, note 2), 110-116.

[4] For a recent analysis, see International Labour Conference 82nd Session 1995, *Report of the Committee of Experts on the Application of Conventions and Recommendations* (Geneva: International Labour Organization, 1995), 107-109.

[5] ARTICLE 19, *State of Fear* (see Chapter 1, note 4), 59.

[6] Burmese Women's Union, *The Plight of Burmese Women* (Bangkok: 1995), 17: Human Rights Watch/Asia, *Burma: Entrenchment or Reform?* (New York: 1995), 14.

[7] Ta Saw Lu, *The Bondage of Opium* (see Chapter 7, note 29), 2-3.

[8] J Boyden, *Myanmar Children in Especially Difficult Circumstances* (Rangoon: UNICEF, 1992), 32.

[9] *National Programme of Action* (see Chapter 2, note 18), 3.

[10] Ibid.

[11] UNICEF, *Children and Women in Myanmar* (see Chapter 2, note 13), 39.

[12] Ibid., at 13. For a rare, independent study of women's health problems in Burma, see F McConville, *A Rapid Participatory Assessment of the Health Needs of Women and Their Children in an Urban Poor Area of Myanmar* (World Vision UK, April-June 1995), which is based on a three month study of 200 mothers in a Rangoon satellite town.

[13] *National Programme of Action*, note 9 above, at 2; UNICEF, note 11 above, at 14.

[14] Ibid. In another calculation, in 1994 UNICEF put Burma's maternal mortality rate even higher — at 460 per 100,000 live births between 1980-1991; see, UNICEF, *The State of the World's Children* (Oxford University Press: 1994), 76.

[15] UNICEF, *Possibilities for a United Nations Peace and Development Initiative* (see Chapter 1, note 2), 2.

[16] UNICEF, note 11 above, at 14-15; the goitre prevalence rate, which is caused by iodine deficiency, is officially put at 28 per cent.

[17] Southeast Asian Information Network, *Out of Control* (see Chapter 7, note 20), 11.

[18] UNICEF, *Country Programme Recommendation: Myanmar* (23 March 1995), Table 1; UNICEF, *Children and Women in Myanmar*, note 11 above, at 16.

[19] Porter, *Wheeling and Dealing* (see Chapter 4, note 18), 69.

[20] UNICEF, note 11 above, at 65.

[21] Ibid., at 38. Fifteen of the young women were below the age of 18.

[22] Human Rights Watch/Asia, *A Modern Form of Slavery* (see Chapter 7, note 5); Smith, note 3 above, at 113-6.

[23] Porter, note 19 above, at 73.

[24] Boyden, note 8 above, at 17.

Chapter 9

THE INTERNATIONAL PERSPECTIVE

Whatever is said publicly, few international organizations — whether inter-governmental or non-governmental — have any illusions about the underlying problems of working in Burma today. As Madeleine Albright, US Permanent Representative to the UN, explained after a recent visit to Burma:

> For years, controversy has surrounded programs conducted within Burma by United Nations agencies, including UNICEF and the UNDP. Their efforts raise a classic policy dilemma: how to help people living under despotism without helping the despots themselves.[1]

For while certain UN bodies, including the UN General Assembly and UN Commission on Human Rights, have persistently investigated and condemned human rights violations by the SLORC, other UN agencies such as the UNDP, UNICEF, WHO and UNHCR continue to try and work inside the country according to their mandates.

Such a policy dilemma has led to considerable debate about the ethics and methods of working within Burma. As the door to Burma slowly opens, international agencies and others have expressed very differing views over the relative merits of various strategies put forward to help foster social and political reform. In particular, a clear division has emerged between those who believe that a policy of "constructive engagement" with the SLORC will help, and those who advocate boycotts and conditionality. Burma's neighbours and some multinational corporations, for example, especially favour an approach of "constructive engagement", while most Burmese opposition parties, human rights groups and governments in the West align in the conditionality or even "boycott" camp. In the meantime, the question of the health rights of the Burmese peoples inevitably becomes hostage to the broader political debate.

In many respects, the UN, international and NGO aid organizations which work on health and development issues in Burma are also divided along these lines. Although it is the political future and health of the Burmese peoples which are at stake, institutional self-interest is undoubtedly a powerful factor. In recent years, the arguments over international aid and development involvement in Burma have become a well-rehearsed subject[2], but experience has shown that discussions over ethics and effective action can quickly degenerate into arguments over a hierarchy of needs. In the process, evidence on a whole array of health and humanitarian issues — from human rights abuses or heroin production to high infant mortality rates and the spread of AIDS — is selectively used by different organizations to produce very different justifications for institutional actions on the health and humanitarian crisis in Burma.

All groups are looking at the same broad body of problems (and, in health matters, share many of the same views), but they often come to describe them in very different terms. Indeed, different international reports in recent years have tended to give the impression that there are two Burmas: one depicted as "Asia's New Killing Fields", where gross human rights violations are endemic, and the other as a belated model of new Asian development, where international agencies working in the country achieve nothing but success.[3] In the latter case, self-censorship plays a critical part in determining the manner in which some agencies present their work, not only so that they will be allowed to continue operations in the country but also, as the imprisonment of the ex-UNICEF researcher Dr Khin Zaw Win has warned, to protect the security of employees who will still be living in Burma long after individual foreign colleagues have gone.

What is actually needed is better mutual understanding of the roles played by medical agencies in the emergency humanitarian field, those working on broader health and development issues, and by those pursuing human rights and political reform without which sustainable development and national health reconstruction are impossible. At the same time, it is essential that the peoples of Burma themselves are able to assert control over their own health destiny.

Nevertheless, a generally-accepted pattern of international intervention in the health field has gradually evolved. Provided that various foreign currency exchange requirements and guarantees of noninterference by the government are met, there is an overall consensus (supported by the European Union and other world bodies) that the situation of refugees and other health emergencies must receive priority attention in the delivery of humanitarian aid, while, for other development assistance, only projects based at the community level are acceptable. This approach underpinned the exceptional decision in Burma's case of the UNDP's Governing Council in May 1992 to begin a review of its country programme so that future work would be limited to critical humanitarian and basic "human development initiatives" at the "grass-roots level".[4] This reorientation was then approved by the UNDP's Governing Council decision 93/21 of June 1993, which strictly demarcated the "human development" areas of work that the decision permits. Since this time, there has been much emphasis amongst both UN and NGO aid organizations working in Burma on such issues as "capacity building", "community development", "community participation", "social mobilization" and "integrated participatory planning at the village/grassroots level" in assessing the sustainability and impact of projects.[5] That health and humanitarian issues are often considered to be separate from issues of political reform and human rights was also reflected in the December 1995 decision of the Japanese government to postpone a scheduled yen loan to Burma "because of stalled efforts to democratize the country" and, instead, use the proposed resumption of aid funding to help build a nursing college in Rangoon.[6]

The key question, however, as to whether such international humanitarian programmes can achieve their goals, remains unanswered. There can be no doubt, for example, that improved clinical skills, modern diagnosis techniques and improved immunization and sanitation programmes will boost the levels of health care for those to whom they are available. Yet, in the view of many, including Burmese opposition groups, until there is substantial political reform in Burma, such projects will remain just a drop in the ocean in terms of health and development needs. Indeed, many medical practitioners believe that an important first step in any health reform programme must be to strengthen and upgrade the delivery capacity of the Health Ministry and public system of national health. This, in any country in the world, is the main line in health defence and co-ordination. Focusing on the grass roots level without also addressing the poor performance of the national system may thus be misguided. Commented one Burmese physician:

> All this talk about communities and NGOs has become a bit of a smokescreen which every side can use. If health standards are really to improve, what is really needed is an integrated approach, where every health agency is energized and health information and techniques are freely shared and acted upon. This simply is not happening at present. Burma is still very socially divided.

Similarly, as Dr David Dapice of the Harvard Institute for International Development recently wrote in a report to the UNDP:

> The current UNDP activities in Myanmar/Burma are strictly limited to grass-roots humanitarian efforts in a widely scattered handful of townships. These bottom-up anti-poverty initiatives have done a great deal of good in these local areas, but clearly fall short of addressing the comprehensive national problems confronting the country. Systematic assistance to national policy is not possible under the current mandate.[7]

Without political reform, then — including guarantees on freedom of information, expression, association and participation — huge doubts must remain about the long-term quality or impact of international initiatives. The protection of such rights presupposes the existence of a strong civil society. For the moment, however, this is lacking in Burma. As Professor David Steinberg, a Burma specialist and representative of the Asia Foundation in Korea, has written: "Burma today effectively has no civil society ... .In a sense the SLORC has been attempting to create its own civil society — one that it controls."[8]

For the present, the SLORC alone determines not only which international organizations can enter the country, but where and how they can work and what supplies or funds they can import and distribute. In October 1994 the SLORC Secretary-One, Lieutenant-General

Khin Nyunt, told a Border Areas Developent Committee meeting that "offers" of assistance from international agencies and NGOs would only be accepted "as long as they do not threaten national security and solidarity". As a result, despite the stated emphasis of international agencies on community-led development, many supporters of the National League for Democracy or ethnic opposition groups claim that they are being excluded from projects under way or under discussion — and are even being prevented from making the same international contacts from inside the country. For example, in an AIDS training course run by World Vision for "community development groups" in Kawthaung, only three groups were represented: the MMCWA, MRC and USDA, all of which are widely perceived to be under the control of the government.[9]

Thus, far from bringing the benefits of health care and grass roots participation to the community, many opposition groups argue that such programmes serve only to strengthen the SLORC and increase its legitimacy. Indeed, such concerns prompted Aung San Suu Kyi to write to Mr Gustave Speth, Administrator of the UNDP, in January 1996 pointing out the discrimination that many ordinary people face in gaining access to aid and requesting that, in future, the "funds, programmes and agencies of the United Nations" should consider ways of implementing projects "in close co-operation with the NLD"; in this way, Suu Kyi argued, UN agencies would be working with the only organization in Burma which, through the result of the 1990 election, has been shown to represent the "will of the people" in accordance with the "principles of the Universal Declaration of Human Rights" and the resolutions on Burma of the UN General Assembly.[10]

The SLORC's immediate response was to launch strong public attacks on Aung San Suu Kyi in the state-controlled media in an apparent attempt to prevent such links between the NLD and international agencies from developing (see Chapter 5). In the United States, meanwhile, where there has long been frustration over the failure of the SLORC to introduce substantive reform, the US Congress proposed legislation to limit any future donations from US voluntary contributions to the UNDP programme in Burma under four strict conditions: that all funded programmes should focus on "eliminating human suffering"; be undertaken only through international or private voluntary organizations that the NLD leadership deems "independent" of the SLORC; provide "no financial, political or military benefit to the SLORC"; and are supported by the NLD.[11]

Burma's political crisis thus continues to impinge on the health field, and the underlying dilemmas for international agencies remain unresolved. But, as Aung San Suu Kyi once explained:

> People's participation in social and political trans-
> formation is the central issue of our time. This can
> only be achieved through the establishment of so-
> cieties which place human worth above power, and
> liberation above control. In this paradigm, devel-
> opment requires democracy, the genuine empow-
> erment of the people.[12]

NOTES

[1] Madeleine Albright, "Burmese Daze", *The New Republic*, 4 Dec. 1995, reproduced in *Burma Debate*, Nov./Dec. 1995, 19.

[2] See e.g., H Yawnghwe, "Engaging the Generals" and M Smith, "Humanitarian and Development Aid to Burma" in *Burma Debate*, July/Aug. 1994, 4-9 and 16-21; World Vision, *The Role of NGOs in Burma* (Milton Keynes: 1995).

[3] For a variety of views, see e.g., A Clements (with a foreword by the Dalai Lama), *Burma: The Next Killing Fields?* (Berkeley: Odonian Press, 1992); World Vision, note 2 above; Agrodev Canada Inc., *UNDP's Myanmar Human Development Initiative* (see Chapter 5, note 15).

[4] UNDP, *Summary Report: UNDP Assistance to Myanmar* (see Chapter 2, note 19); Agrodev Canada, note 3 above, at 2. In line with these goals, the UNDP targeted such basic health and development areas as primary health, malaria, HIV/AIDS and water-supply projects.

[5] See e.g., ibid., at 2-9; World Vision, *Report on Review of the AIDS Awareness, Education and Prevention Project in Kawthaung* (see Chapter 7, note 20), 1-2. In January 1996, despite letters of protest from the NLD (see below), the Governing Council of the UNDP decided to approve a further full five-year programme for Burma.

[6] *Daily Yomiuri*, 13 Dec. 1995.

[7] Dapice, *Prospects for Sustainable Growth* (see Chapter 4, note 11), 2.

[8] D Steinberg, "Civil Society in Burma", *Forum of Democratic Leaders in the Asia Pacific Region Quarterly*, Winter 1995, 7.

[9] World Vision, note 5 above, at 5.

[10] Letter, Aung San Suu Kyi, General-Secretary of the NLD, to Gustave Speth, Administrator of the UNDP, 14 Jan. 1996. Copies of this letter, and a subsequent letter dated 26 Feb. 1996, were later widely circulated.

[11] House of Representatives, *Conference Report: Foreign Relations Authorization Act, Fiscal Years 1996 and 1997* (Washington, 104th Congress, 5 March 1996), 46-47. See also, Chapter 7, note 32.

[12] Daw Aung San Suu Kyi, *Empowerment for a Culture of Peace and Development*, address to the World Commission on Culture and Development, Manila, 21 Nov. 1994, delivered by Corazon Aquino.

Chapter 10

CONCLUSIONS AND RECOMMENDATIONS

A s this report shows, Burma today faces not just a political impasse which calls out for world attention but a public health crisis of enormous and worsening proportions, which partly stems from years of military misrule. Elsewhere, such crises affecting the health of a nation may arise from climatic or other natural factors, or the impact of particular cultural values or religious practices. But Burma's health crisis is man-made — the product of long years of political isolation and ethnic conflict, widespread repression and human rights violations, and a continuing official obsession with secrecy and censorship. The public's right to know about all manner of issues vital to the enjoyment of their basic rights, including the right to health, has been subordinated to the political survival of an undemocratic military elite at what can only be described as incalculable cost.

Today, eight years after the SLORC seized power and brutally suppressed the democracy movement, there are signs that the ruling elite has recognized the crisis breaking around it and sees the need for some remedial action, even at the cost of allowing a degree of international involvement in Burma's affairs. International agencies and NGOs are now increasingly being allowed into Burma, though under strictly controlled conditions, and at the economic level, the SLORC is pursuing an avowedly "open door" policy to encourage international investment. These will be welcome developments if, in fact, they represent a real recognition of the need for, and a genuine commitment to change. This, however, is still uncertain.

What is clear is that efforts in the direction of reform, including greater protection of the health rights of the peoples of Burma, will come to nothing unless freedom of expression and the right to information — the public's right to know — are also assured. Currently, free and open discussion about issues central to individual and family health, and debate as to how these can best be resolved, is simply not possible under the strict censorship regime enforced by the SLORC. Likewise, the state's monopoly over information and its propensity to tailor official statistics for political purposes, together with continuing curbs on access to particular areas of the country, mean that doctors, scientists and others are denied crucial information relating to public health, and are thus ill-equipped to respond to what should be priority needs.

Burma's burgeoning health crisis, in ARTICLE 19's view, requires a political as well as a medical response. Health rights cannot be ensured in isolation, just as Burma's economic woes cannot be addressed without recourse to fundamental political change — change which ensures popular participation in decision-making and true government accountability, none of which can occur without freedom of expression, public access to information and effective protection of other human rights.

There is a need for the international community as a whole to help the Burmese peoples address the many problems and challenges that confront them. This has been long recognized within the international community itself, as evidenced by successive UN resolutions on Burma, the involvement in Burma of UN and other international agencies, and by the assistance made available by local and international NGOs to refugees from the conflicts in Burma. Today, as the SLORC tentatively seeks to open up Burma to the wider world, there are real opportunities for governments to exert a positive influence, if they have the will to do so. In particular, the SLORC is currently negotiating Burma's entry into ASEAN and it is seeking significant inward investment not only from its Asian neighbours and Japan but also from the countries of the West, including the European Union and the United States. The governments of these countries must make it clear to the SLORC that human rights are universal and indivisible, and that closer and mutually-beneficial relations with Burma cannot be achieved unless there is rapid, irreversible and fundamental reform in Burma itself. They should do this singly, in their bilateral relations with the SLORC, and in unison as part of a united international front for the restoration of human rights and democracy in Burma. Any failure to do so will be no less than to acquiesce in prolonging the suffering of the peoples of Burma.

Sustained international concern, economic and political pressure are all key to bringing change in Burma. For this reason, ARTICLE 19 urges governments around the world, especially those maintaining close relations with the SLORC, to endorse and support the agenda for reform set out below.

Yet, the primary responsibility lies with those currently holding power in Rangoon. It is they and their military predecessors, very largely, who have presided over Burma's decline to its present parlous state, and it is they who have the most particular obligation now to initiate effective reform.

ARTICLE 19 is, therefore, calling on the SLORC to take the following, urgent steps to address both the health crisis now besetting Burma and the political and human rights wrongs which so very largely brought it about:

• To release immediately and unconditionally all prisoners and detainees held on account of their peaceful exercise of the right to freedom of expression, including Dr Ma Thida, Dr Khin Zaw Win, Dr Zaw Myint, Dr Zaw Myint Maung and other members of the medical profession, and to end the threats made against Aung San Suu Kyi and other democracy leaders in the state-controlled media.

• To cease immediately torture and other human rights violations which directly affect the health of the victims or their families; to bring to justice all those responsible for torture or other grave human rights violations; and to compensate the victims and their families.

• To end the use of forced labour, including of porters for the military, and other state practices which harm or threaten individual health rights.

• To lift the blanket of censorship currently in place and to guarantee, in law and practice, the right to freedom of expression and access to information, including about vital issues affecting individual and family health, such as the right to reproductive health information.

• To remove all restrictions on freedom of movement, association and assembly and to foster the development of independent, indigenous NGOs as a means of facilitating the widest possible participation in the elaboration of health policy, research, training and public education about health issues.

• To give particular attention to the health needs of women and other vulnerable or marginalized groups, including children, members of ethnic and religious minorities, the disabled, and returning refugees and displaced peoples.

• To reinstate all medical practitioners and health workers dismissed or excluded from pursuing their profession on account of their political beliefs.

• To allow medical practitioners, academics, writers and others to research and report on health issues in Burma free from censorship or restrictions on freedom of association and movement. The authorities should ensure the widest possible dissemination within Burma of all research and other pertinent information on health and humanitarian issues, including the results of investigations by local researchers as well as that undertaken by international humanitarian and other agencies.

• To ensure open access to all parts of the country to journalists, as well as to local and international academic and other researchers, in order to investigate matters of humanitarian and human rights concern. No obstacles should be placed on the free flow of information on such issues.

• To ensure that the health rights of all prisoners and others held in custody are fully protected; that all deaths in custody are promptly and impartially investigated; and that all prisoners are treated in accordance with the UN Standard Minimum Rules for the Treatment of Prisoners.

• To invite the International Committee of the Red Cross (ICRC) to resume operations in Burma, by guaranteeing the ICRC unfettered and regular access to all prisons and prisoners, including all those held on security grounds or taken prisoner in the course of conflict, in accordance with the ICRC's standard requirements for access to prisoners.

• To cease all offensive military operations, allow humanitarian assistance to victims of conflict, and comply with UN General Assembly demands to commence a process of "substantive political dialogue...with Aung San Suu Kyi and other political leaders, including representatives from ethnic groups, as the best means of promoting national reconciliation and the full and early restoration of democracy."

• To sign and ratify key international treaties relating to the protection and promotion of human rights, in particular those listed below, and to amend existing law and practice to ensure full conformity with these instruments:

— the International Covenant on Civil and Political Rights and its (first) Optional Protocol;

— the International Covenant on Economic, Social and Cultural Rights;

— the Convention against Torture and Other Cruel, Inhuman or Degrading Treatment or Punishment;

— the Convention on the Elimination of All Forms of Discrimination against Women;

— the Convention relating to the Status of Refugees.

SELECTED BIBLIOGRAPHY

Agrodev Canada Inc., *UNDP's Myanmar Human Development Initiative: An Assessment* (Ottawa: 1995).

ARTICLE 19, *The Right to Know: Human Rights and Access to Reproductive Health Information* (London and Philadelphia: ARTICLE 19 and University of Pennsylvania Press, 1995).

ARTICLE 19, *Censorship Prevails: Political Deadlock and Economic Transition in Burma* (London: 1995).

ARTICLE 19, *Starving in Silence: A Report on Famine and Censorship* (London: 1990).

Burmese Border Consortium, *Refugee Relief Programme: Programme Report for Period January to June 1995* (Bangkok: 1995).

Human Rights Watch, *Indivisible Human Rights: The Relationship of Political and Civil Rights to Survival, Subsistence and Poverty* (New York: 1992).

Human Rights Watch/Asia - *A Modern Form of Slavery: Trafficking of Burmese Women and Girls into Brothels in Thailand* (New York: 1993).

Médecins Sans Frontières, *Populations in Danger 1995* (London: 1995).

Médecins Sans Frontières, *MSF's Concerns on the Repatriation of Rohingya Refugees from Bangladesh to Burma* (Amsterdam and Paris: MSF, 1995).

Physicians for Human Rights, *Health and Human Rights in Burma (Myanmar)* (Boston: 1991).

Milton Roemer, *Primary Health Care in Burma's National Health System* (Rangoon: Western Consortium for the Health Professions and United States Agency for International Development, 1986).

Martin Smith, *Ethnic Groups in Burma: Development, Democracy and Human Rights* (London: Anti-Slavery International, 1994).

Southeast Asian Information Network, *Out of Control: the HIV/AIDS Epidemic in Burma* (Chiang Mai: December 1995).

UNHCR, *Return to Myanmar: Repatriating Refugees from Bangladesh* (Information Bulletin, June 1995).

UNICEF, *Children and Women in Myanmar: A Situation Analysis 1995* (Rangoon: 1995).

Union of Myanmar, *National Health Plan: 1993-1996* (Rangoon: Ministry of Health).

World Bank, *Myanmar: Policies for Sustaining Economic Reform* (New York: 1995).

World Vision, *The Role of NGOs in Burma* (Milton Keynes: 1995).

SELECTED ARTICLE 19
PUBLICATIONS

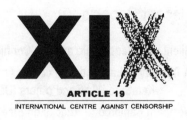

ARTICLE 19
INTERNATIONAL CENTRE AGAINST CENSORSHIP

Books

The Right to Know - Human Rights and Access to Reproductive Health
Information (Aug.1995) 416pp., £18.00/$30.00

La Liberté de la Presse et de l'information au Maroc - limites et perspectives
(Joint report with OMDH,June 1995) 360pp. £5.99/$8.0, available from
OMDH Morocco

Who Rules the Airwaves? Broadcasting in Africa (March 1995) 168pp.,
£9.99/$15.00

Fiction, Fact and the *Fatwa*: 2,000 Days of Censorship (Aug. 1994) 190pp.,
£7.95/$15.00

Guidelines for Election Broadcasting in Transitional Democracies (Aug. 1994)
124pp., £9.99/$15.00

Forging War: The Media in Serbia, Croatia and Bosnia-Hercegovina (May 1994)
288pp., £9.99/$15.00

Freedom of Expression Handbook: International and Comparative Law,
Standards and Procedures (Aug. 1993) 322pp., £12.00/$20.00

Press Law and Practice: A Comparative Study of Press Freedom in European
and Other Democracies (April 1993) 320pp., £12.00/$20.00

Striking a Balance: Hate Speech, Freedom of Expression and Non-Discrimination
(May 1992) 432pp., £9.95/$15.00

State of Fear: Censorship in Burma (Dec. 1991) 120pp., £3.95/$6.00

Starving in Silence: A Report on Famine and Censorship (April 1990) 146pp.,
£3.95/$6.00

Recent Reports

Silent War: Censorship and the Conflict in Sri Lanka (March 1996) £3.99/$6.00

A Travesty of Law and Justice: An Analysis of the Judgement in the Case of Ken Saro-Wiwa and others (Dec. 1995) 23pp., £3.99/$6.00

Northern Cameroon - Attacks on Freedom of Expression by Governmental and Traditional Authorities (July 1995) 36pp., £3.00/$5.00

Nigeria - Fundamental Human Rights Denied: Report of the Trial of Ken Saro-Wiwa and Others (June 1995) 36pp., £3.00/$6.00

Broken Promises - Freedom of Expression in Hong Kong (Joint Report with the Hong Kong Journalists Association, June 1995) 40pp., £3.00/$5.00

Censorship in Kenya: Government Critics Face the Death Sentence (March 1995) 40pp., £3.99/$6.00

Censorship Prevails: Political Deadlock and Economic Transition in Burma (March 1995) 60pp., £3.99/$6.00

An Agenda for Change: The Right to Freedom of Expression in Sri Lanka (Oct. 1994) 64pp., £4.99/$10.00

Censorship News Reports

MOZAMBIQUE: Freedom of Expression and "The Vote for Peace" (Oct. 1995)

INDONESIA: Surveillance and Suppression - The Legacy of the 1965 Coup (Sept. 1995)

INDONESIA: The Press on Trial (Aug. 1995)

SRI LANKA: Words into Action - Censorship and Media Reform (March 1995)

ALGERIA: Secret Decree - New Attack on the Media (Nov. 1994)

GAMBIA: Democracy Overturned - Violations of Freedom of Expression (Dec. 1994)

MOZAMBIQUE: Freedom of Expression and the Elections (Oct. 1994)

MALAWI: Freedom of Expression - The Elections and the Need for Media Reform (July 1994)

MALAWI's Elections: Media Monitoring, Freedom of Expression and Intimidation (April 1994)

JORDAN: Democratization without Press Freedom (March 1994)

ALGERIA: Assassination in the Name of Religion (Dec. 1993)

TUNISIA: The Press in Tunisia - Plus ça change (Nov. 1993)

MALAWI's Past: The Right to Truth (Nov. 1993)

KENYA: Shooting the Messenger (Oct. 1993)

SUDAN: Dismantling Civil Society - Suppression of Freedom of Association
(Aug. 1993)

Bulletin

The ARTICLE 19 Newsletter, published 3 times per year. The Bulletin is available for an annual subscription of £15/US$25 which includes membership.

Subscriptions

An Annual Subscription to all ARTICLE 19 publications is available at a cost including postage of £75 (UK) or £85/US$130 (Overseas).

Please add the following to your payment for postage and packing:

UK and EC countries - Orders under £25/US$40 add 20% of total; orders over £25, add 10%.

Overseas - add 50% of total for airmail; 20% for surface mail.

*** Only cheques drawn in UK £ sterling or US dollars can be accepted.***

All publications are available from:

ARTICLE 19
The International Centre Against Censorship

33 Islington High Street, London N1 9LH, United Kingdom
Tel: (0171) 278 9292 Fax: (0171) 713 1356
E-mail: article19@gn.apc.org

Trade Distribution:
Central Books
99 Wallis Road, London, E9 5LN
Tel: 0181-986 4854 Fax: 0181-533 5821

ARTICLE 19

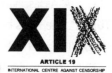

The International Centre Against Censorship

ARTICLE 19 takes its name and purpose from Article 19 of the Universal Declaration of Human Rights.

Everyone has the right to freedom of opinion and expression; this right includes freedom to hold opinions without interference and to seek, receive and impart information and ideas through any media and regardless of frontiers.

ARTICLE 19 works impartially and systematically to oppose censorship worldwide. We work on behalf of victims of censorship — individuals who are physically attacked, killed, unjustly imprisoned, restricted in their movements or dismissed from their jobs; print and broadcast media which are censored, banned or threatened; organizations, including political groups or trades unions, which are harassed, suppressed or silenced.

ARTICLE 19's programme of research, publication, campaign and legal intervention addresses censorship in its many forms. We monitor individual countries' compliance with international standards protecting the right to freedom of expression and work at the governmental and inter-governmental level to promote greater respect for this fundamental right.

ARTICLE 19 has established a growing international network of concerned individuals and organizations who promote awareness of censorship issues and take action on individual cases.

ARTICLE 19 is a non-governmental organization, entirely dependent on donations (UK Charity No. 327421). For more information contact:

ARTICLE 19

Lancaster House, 33 Islington High Street, London N1 9LH
Tel: 0171 278 9292 Fax: 0171 713 1356, E-mail: article19@gn.apc.org